Religions, Culture and Healthcare

Second Edition

Religions, Culture and Healthcare

A practical handbook for use in healthcare environments

Second Edition

Susan Hollins
NHS Chaplain and Life Coach

Radcliffe Publishing
Oxford • New York

Radcliffe Publishing Ltd
18 Marcham Road
Abingdon
Oxon OX14 1AA
United Kingdom

www.radcliffe-oxford.com
Electronic catalogue and worldwide online ordering facility.

British Library Cataloguing in Publication Data

A catalogue record for this book is available from the British Library.

ISBN-13 978 1 84619 260 9

Typeset by Anne Joshua & Associates, Oxford
Printed and bound by TJI Digital, Padstow, Cornwall

Contents

Foreword to the first edition

It is with great pleasure that I write this foreword for *Religions, Culture and Healthcare: a practical handbook for use in healthcare environments.* In the Equality and Human Rights Group at the Department of Health, we actively promote innovative approaches to embedding the principles of equality, fair treatment, dignity and respect and valuing diversity into the Department and the NHS. These values and principles lie at the heart of the Department's drive to recognise the needs of patients and staff from diverse religious groups, and to respond sensitively and appropriately to those needs.

This is a much-welcomed guide on an issue which is at the heart of so many of us – our faith, our individual cultural identity, and our religious and spiritual needs. We are fortunate to live in a multi-cultural, multi-faith society, and the fact that the UK has more diverse faith communities than any other country in the European Union is something that we have every reason to be proud of. Valuing differences unites us, bringing us together and strengthening our society.

This guidance highlights the importance of celebrating this diversity as well as dealing with the challenges it poses us. It promotes a commitment to dignity and respect, to providing appropriate and sensitive care to all, and to patient-led care and individual choice at all stages of a patient's health and social care, from birth to the end of life.

It is a key part of the NHS Plan that any reform of the NHS and social care must ensure the delivery of fair, appropriate and equitable access of services to all. Indeed, the White Paper *Choosing Health*, published in November 2004, underlined our aim for everyone to achieve improved health, and to focus specifically on inequalities in health.

Spiritual care, then, is something that is essential within the NHS. As an organisation employing over 1.4 million staff, and with over five and a half million elective hospital admissions every year, it's vital that the NHS positions itself at the forefront of recognising the needs of the diverse patients and users that are part of, and use, its services.

We need to ensure that we are able to respond to the religious and spiritual needs of patients and staff, whatever their faith or belief. This is why I am delighted to write the foreword for this guidance which contributes towards making the NHS a place where people from all backgrounds feel valued, respected and treated fairly – a crucial goal for us all in delivering a patient-led NHS.

Surinder Sharma
National Director for Equality and Human Rights
Department of Health and the NHS
December 2005

Preface to the second edition

All healthcare providers are required to have a sound working knowledge of the main religions to enable them to give sensitive and appropriate care to patients. This handbook is intended to be of practical assistance to healthcare staff in helping them to gain a fuller understanding of the nine world faiths and to be able to apply this knowledge in a variety of circumstances. I have also included information about some less well-known and some emerging faith communities as these also take their place within a society where diversity is the norm and no longer the exception. Collectively these faith communities represent a cultural and religious diversity that is vibrant and creative. Individually they may present challenges to healthcare providers to develop and manage their services in ways that are more sensitive and responsive to their patients' particular needs.

A major precept in this book, both explicit and implicit, is the necessity for healthcare professionals to maintain an openness of mind – a positive regard – towards all patients, and to seek to avoid at all costs an easy placing of them within certain stereotypical frames. In this way the care that is provided can be of the highest order in relation to the patients' cultural, religious and spiritual needs and requirements. The information provided here could be regarded as a starting point on a journey of mutual discovery between the healthcare provider and the patient. On this journey into new territory there are highly significant clues to inform and improve not only the relationship between the healthcare professional and the patient, but also to improve the outcome of treatment.

The design of this handbook is intended to facilitate access to various types of information relating to the different stages and needs of life from within the spectrum of both major and minor religions. It is not intended that it should sit on a high shelf behind the locked doors of an office. Better that it is always to be found, increasingly dog-eared perhaps, at the nursing station, and in the pockets of doctors and other non-ward-based healthcare staff. Although it has been my intention to provide essential and relevant information, I have steered away from an encyclopaedic approach. I hope that as healthcare professionals gather this essential information they will also become confident in its judicious application, avoiding the stereotypical responses in order to discover the individual at the heart of their care. If additional information about certain aspects of patient care within a particular religion is needed, I hope that the Resources section at the end of the volume will provide further signposts for this journey.

Susan Hollins
January 2009

About the author

Following 16 years as a priest in the parochial ministry of The Church of England, Susan Hollins has worked in the UK National Health Service as a healthcare chaplain since 1999, firstly in the acute sector, followed in 2004 by work at national level developing a workforce strategy for NHS healthcare chaplains. She is the author of a new and extremely comprehensive list of religious affiliations and belief systems which is to be used extensively in the UK National Health Service and government organisations. Trained in psychodynamic counselling and following a recent appointment at the Royal Brompton Hospital in London Susan now works as a life coach.

Acknowledgements

Much of the information contained within this book is in the public domain, and is often passed on by word of mouth. My role therefore has been that of gatherer of scattered information. Other people have also been collecting this important information for use not only within healthcare, but also in business environments in our globally diverse community.

Dedication

For my Father – a true seeker on his winding spiritual journey – remembering you with love and gratitude.

Chapter I

Cultural and religious diversity within healthcare

Who am I? I am not the sum total of clinical statistics held on my health record. I am not 'Bed 27 CA breast (or whatever illness I might happen to have).' When I come into your hospital as a patient, I may feel like a stranger in a foreign land. I do not speak *'clinical-ese'* or *'medical-itian.'* I may not know how to get to the ward or the unit without the need for signposts, verbal directions and the hospital map, now deeply creased with greasy patches held tightly in my rather moist hand. I feel vulnerable. I feel naked even though I am wearing my clothes (or some of them). By contrast, you may seem to me like some foreign force who, with knives and machines and other alien implements, may threaten to invade the land that is my body and cause overwhelming feelings of fear and anxiety to wash over me like waves breaking on a beach in a storm. Whatever my physical or mental condition when I arrive in your territory, you may have your way, and I will give my consent, perhaps unwillingly yet knowingly, bartering and negotiating my way through the minefield of procedures until I catch sight of the door marked Exit – and, gaining your consent, am given my discharge papers and sight of the door to my home.

Although this might be a rather exaggerated (and vividly imagined!) narrative of a patient experience in any hospital, nevertheless it seeks to capture some of the strong feelings of anxiety, apprehension and even hostility that many patients experience when they enter hospital either as emergency admissions or as elective patients. Yet if my language and my cultural, religious and spiritual maps and compass are not set in the same way as yours, if the way that I dress seems to hide who I am and risks frustrating your professional care, we may as a result be at cross-purposes and I may be the loser.

Hospitals are foreign territories, and they remain so despite the increase in sensitive and patient-friendly health design in many parts of the world. This patient-friendly design seeks to soften and domesticate the real and necessary business of healthcare which, although multifaceted, is necessarily clinical, and may often feel immensely impersonal despite the soft facades and all the other well-intentioned strategies to assist my journey through this new-found strange land.

Healthcare staff may forget that, to begin with at least, they may be regarded as members of the invading force, the alien enemy, even though their task and calling is high and healing. Healthcare staff have a crucial role in setting the patient at ease in this foreign territory. They are the welcoming party who sues for peace. They are the translators of *clinical-ese* and *medical-itian* into everyday language so that the patient and his or her relatives may understand the process and procedures. They are the givers of reassurance alongside the medication. They are the astute communicators between the patient and other healthcare staff. Their understanding of what it feels to be ill, vulnerable and scared needs to be profound. As providers of 'hospital-ity', they recognise that their patients are also customers – key stakeholders in a multi-billion-dollar business. We are all in the numbers game after all, or so it seems . . .

But what does all of this have to do with cultural and religious diversity? It has everything to do with the culturally diverse societies in which we live. Religion still plays a key part – both conscious and unconscious – in the social identity of individuals, communities and neighbourhoods. Unless we are able to appreciate and understand that hidden within the long robes of the Muslim woman, under the Kippah of an Orthodox Jewish man, within the seasonal rituals practised by the young Wiccan or in the family photos arranged on the top of the bedside locker there are major clues to the mystery of the person in the bed, then caring for patients of all cultures – the obvious and the hidden – will remain a game of clinical and financial numbers.

Hospitals are places where people struggle to hang on to their individuality amid the clinical procedures set in place to help to restore their mental and/or physical health. Failing to pay adequate attention to the individual only reinforces their vulnerability and a perception that they are no longer in control of what happens to them, despite the consent forms that they are required to sign.

It is no secret that the populations of Western Europe and the USA are becoming increasingly diverse. For example, in the USA, by 2050 the number of adults belonging to what are now termed minority ethnic groups (Hispanic, Black, Asian, Native American, Native Hawaiian, Pacific Islander or Mixed Race) is projected to be 439 million or 54% of the total adult population. The Hispanic adult population alone is projected to increase to 133 million or 30% of the total population. By contrast, the proportion of Non-Hispanic Whites in the adult population is projected to decrease from the current level of 66% to 46% over the same time period.[1]

It has become normative for people to respond in non-religious terms when invited to state whether they have any religious affiliation on admission to hospital. In so many ways the term 'spiritual, but not religious' captures the freeing up of people's thinking and believing in relation to the traditional and ancient faiths that have spanned thousands of years. In the USA, where religion exercises considerable influence at all levels of public and private life, the Religious Landscape Forum Survey indicates a marked and noteworthy increase (16%) in the number of Americans who state that they are unaffiliated to any particular religion.

Diversity and fluidity are now key words in any discussion, debate and decision making about the provision and delivery of healthcare services. The reason for this is that cultural diversity has become a permanent characteristic of our western societies, even if our national institutions, government bodies, and private businesses and local communities are to a greater or lesser extent playing 'catch-up' with this reality. Diversity is also the pacemaker specifically in relation to the increasing fluidity of people's religious affiliation and sense of belonging to a particular faith. As cultural diversity increases and deepens in our common life, so other religions and spiritual pathways present themselves to us for consideration. We may regard cultural and religious diversity as colours in a giant palette of paints – so many shades and nuances of colour from which we may choose, to a greater or lesser extent, the particular colours for our own lives. Whereas religious belief among members of families was once set firm, and was handed on from generation to generation, the current patterns of religious affiliation now reveal far greater fluidity, flux and change. People now feel at greater liberty to choose a different faith from the one in which they were nurtured within their family. Among families it is more common for there to be members of more than one particular faith, as well as members who do not have or do not wish to have a specific faith. What seems to be emerging is a gradual shift from a religion-centric life to a spirituality-centric life. Within Western society as a whole, then, it seems fair to say that people's regard for their lives is understood far more in terms of a spiritual journey of discovery that encompasses the whole of life, with many twists and turns along the way, than in terms of a straight road marked by certainties.

In the American Religious Identification Survey (ARIS Survey) 2001, respondents were asked 'What is your religion, if any?'[2] The replies revealed a significant difference between respondents who identified with a particular religion and those who were affiliated to one. The authors of the ARIS Survey describe it in the following terms: 'identification as a state of heart and mind and affiliation as a social condition.'[2] So it is that respondents in both the ARIS Survey and the Pew Forum Survey spoke of identifying with a particular religion even though their attendance at a place of worship might be irregular (i.e. on a broad spectrum encompassing complete non-attendance, monthly attendance and irregular attendance). What mattered most to these respondents was that they identified with a particular religion even though they rarely worshipped with other members of the same faith community. The factors that give rise to this feeling of identification with a particular religion will of course be immensely varied.

We know that stereotypes reinforce negative thoughts about those who are different from ourselves, yet how often do we base our approach to patients upon such stereotypes? How often do we work from the foundation of our own assumptions and limited knowledge about other cultures and traditions when caring for patients? Such limited knowledge and understanding only serve to reduce the quality of care that we provide for those whose language, lifestyle and belief system are clearly different from our own.

We are cultural beings. From birth to death, culture informs and shapes us – for better as well as for worse. Every culture has its shadow side, which often emerges at times of personal or communal crisis, when we discover its limitations. The positive elements of our culture are often what we recall when we are far from what we recognise as our home and our roots, and when we crave the familiarity and comfort of what is normal and usual to us in terms of the food we eat, the language we use, the buildings we inhabit and the things we enjoy doing. Between the crisis and the need for 'home comfort', culture is implicit in every part of our lives, so that it may become impossible to define what is culturally distinct about ourselves and the community that we call 'ours.' Sometimes definitions and critiques of our culture belong only to the comedian and the satirist, or to the travel writer – those who enjoy observing the oddities and richness of what is usual and ordinary, and commenting upon them in their idiosyncratic ways that make us laugh or rage, or both. Within a society that is inherently diverse, we can no longer live as if the culture is monochrome. Even within societies that share a common heritage and language, there are cultural nuances and shifts, so that we are identified by our regional accents, the phrases that we use at particular times, the food we eat and the clothes we choose to wear. These straightforward examples of cultural diversity illustrate a simple truth, namely that societies have been both threatened and strengthened by rich diversity throughout history. We also know, at great cost, that cultures and whole peoples have been destroyed by an unbalanced desire on the part of others for a monochrome culture that can be controlled. In many countries today there is a far greater diversity of people from vastly different cultures who seek to coexist creatively and to build a future together. One of the essential characteristics of membership of such a society is that each of us has a responsibility not only to understand our own culture but also to discover and understand other cultures. There is a requirement for us all to become far more literate about cultures that are different from our own. In embarking upon a journey of discovery about other cultures, the oppor- tunity to grow in tolerance and understanding towards others who are 'not like us' presents itself very clearly. Within healthcare environments, where patients are naturally vulnerable, our greater understanding and appreciation of different cultures will deepen our pastoral care as well as our clinical care.

The image of an onion, with many different layers, has been used to describe the different elements within a cultural identity.[3] The different layers illustrate the ways in which culture influences our lives, from the implicit to the explicit. The outer layer illustrates how culture influences the outward, external elements of our lives (e.g. the food we eat, the design of the buildings in our towns and cities). The second layer illustrates how culture informs and shapes the norms and values in our society and community. At this level the influences are often unspoken and implicit, tending towards universal themes which relate to ethical standards and values. The final, core layer contains those elements of culture whose threads can be traced through centuries of evolution and development. These also focus upon the initial creation and foundation of a community, and ultimately a civilisation – the immediate environment, and the potential resources of climate and geography for the establishment and maintenance of a society. It is this deeply hidden element or layer of culture that provides the foundation for the other layers that emerge over time as the society matures and develops. It is this core element that provides the 'basic assumptions' of any culture,[3] which are deeply implicit and not generally articulated.

Gert Hofstede, the Dutch cultural analyst, has identified several levels of uniqueness in what he terms 'human mental programming.'[4] These levels of uniqueness are *human nature* (the foundation level), *culture* (the middle level) and *personality* (the top level). There are also three other key elements that are relevant to each level, namely the universal, that which is inherited, and that which is specific to a particular individual or group. The foundation level of human nature possesses universal characteristics such as needs and wide-ranging abilities, including the ability to feel and express or withhold emotion. These sit alongside inherited characteristics that influence and modify these universal abilities. In the same way, culture is both learned and specific to a group or society. As culture is learned, it is passed not only from one generation to the next, but also between different groups. A person has the capacity to absorb both the learned and the inherited ways of being and interacting in the world and in relationship to others, while possessing unique personal characteristics. This pattern illustrates the fact that human beings have a tremendous capacity to adapt to new and diverse cultural environments and to move between them successfully.

I hope that any broad definition of culture would include the beliefs, values, customs, thoughts, actions and communications both of individuals and of the institutions of racial, ethnic, social or religious groups.[5] This breadth of definition highlights the inherent complexity within culture and reminds us of the requirement to begin to look at life from a perspective other than our own – or, as the Native American saying goes, 'Walk a mile in another man's moccasins before you criticise him.' Yet culture, although multi-layered in itself, is only one element of our complex social identity. These different elements can be seen as fluid or overlapping patterns (*see* Figure 1.1).

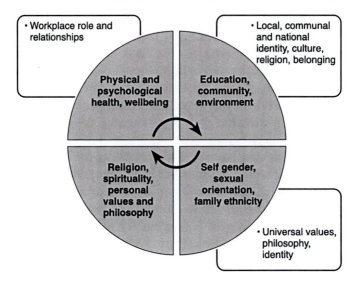

Figure 1.1 Cultural matrix.

From the moment of our birth we are shaped by our experiences, which are set within a familial group, a neighbourhood, a society, a particular religion perhaps, a culture, and an ethnic group. When viewed in this way it is clear that any combination of these elements will provide the dominant strands of our own social identity. So, too, the dominance of any of these elements will shift in relation to the different roles that we undertake. When a person becomes a hospital patient, the pattern shifts once more. Identity then tends to be more focused upon mental and physical health, and upon our primary relationships. Religious and spiritual needs also tend to increase in importance during this time.

Given this varied and fluid pattern, the application of stereotypes is unhelpful. When we attend with interest to just one of the elements that make up another's sense of identity, we begin to enter their world and to see through their eyes. We become more able to recognise the appropriateness – or otherwise – of the care that we provide.

Different cultural traditions also influence the way in which a person will respond to illness and to treatment. Such responses may be as conditioned as those relating to the way in which we dress and behave. Some will regard illness as having a spiritual dimension, sometimes received as a 'judgement' or as some effect of an unknown cause, and they will seek spiritual guidance and support. Others may regard illness as being caused by a combination of several factors, such as lifestyle, environmental conditions, or just bad luck. It is appropriate to take seriously the person's value and belief system as an inherent element within their total care, not only in terms of paying them close attention, but also to support them in tapping into their inner resources and other support networks to strengthen their well-being.

Not everyone has the same attitude towards healthcare professionals. Whereas in western society doctors are held in particularly high regard, in other cultures healthcare staff are regarded as equals, and sometimes as friends in whom one can confide. With such differences in approach and emphasis, it is all the more important for healthcare staff to work towards a mutual understanding of roles and responsibilities with the patients in their care, and to avoid the status quo approach.

Increasing numbers of people have multiple ethnic and cultural identities. In general, people manage to live with these differences and to move smoothly between the different worlds that they represent. However, some people from immigrant communities find the transition from one culture to another so traumatic and destabilising that their mental health suffers. Yet a great deal can be learned from people belonging to minority ethnic groups who have left behind the relative security of their own country with its particular habits and traditions, and who have struggled to adapt to a new and very different – if not alien – culture. During the process of adaptation, which varies in length from one person to another, many people become far more aware of their own culture as well as the new culture. Sometimes this leads them to become more critically aware of the shortcomings of their normative culture at the same time as being critical of the new culture, which may often feel overwhelming. This experience is both costly and potentially creative.

A healthcare culture may threaten to overwhelm the individual patient and their family. This pattern is exacerbated when the culture and ethnic identity of the patient and their relatives differs from that of the country that is providing the healthcare. Immense barriers of language and interpretation are erected, across which the easiest route to take is the normative one, often to the detriment of the patient's well-being. Yet the dominant healthcare culture of a country may also threaten to overwhelm those for whom there are no immediate cultural differences of language. One reason for this is that becoming a hospital patient can be both an alien experience and an alienating one. We are uprooted from all that is familiar in order to become dependent on both the healthcare professionals who treat us and the actual treatment processes that are set in place for our recovery. Adjustment to this change takes time, even when there are no significant cultural barriers. It takes much longer, and may not occur at all, when the cultural differences remain unrecognised to a significant extent. Sometimes a patient may feel that the institution and those who represent it are not heeding their needs and wishes. When this happens, the temptation is for the institution to be defensively inflexible and thus risk losing the remaining trust of the patient.

Culture and language may influence a matrix of elements:

- the way in which illness, disease and their causes are perceived by the patient
- the behaviour of patients, and their attitudes towards healthcare providers
- the delivery of services by the provider, who may not appreciate or understand the cultural traditions and requirements of the patient
- the patient's belief systems with regard to health, well-being and healing.

A variety of cultural competency tools are now available[6] which can be used in healthcare settings to enable deeper and clearer knowledge and understanding about the psychosocial and spiritual needs of patients from different cultures. When used flexibly, these tools help the patient to understand that you are 'on side' with them in seeking to treat them appropriately and with due regard for their spiritual and cultural disposition. In addition, we may develop our own inner checklist of good practice behaviours, an example of which is given below.

- Develop a good awareness and understanding of your own cultural patterns and assumptions, especially where these might inhibit your positive response to patients who have a different culture, religion or lifestyle.
- Be aware that cultural identity is fluid and organic rather than rigid and unchanging.
- Seek to listen to the patient with an open and attentive mind.
- Seek to discover more about the patient's values, beliefs and culture and the ways in which these are important and meaningful to them.
- Seek to avoid stereotypical thinking.
- Maintain an awareness of the other elements that may inform and sustain a person's identity.
- Use information about a person's culture, religion, etc. judiciously, rather than applying it rigorously and without due regard for their individual needs.

Any substantive attention to cultural and religious needs incurs financial costs, such as the provision of adequate interpreting services, or ensuring that sufficient female doctors are employed within a hospital, to take two obvious examples. Yet the financial costs to the health provider tend to be greater when culturally sensitive services are not provided. These costs manifest themselves as formal complaints, to which could be added the psychological cost to the patient and their family. Other elements of cost tend to remain hidden. These include the wasting of both staff and patient time, together with feelings of frustration, helplessness, and disillusion, alienation and a failure of trust among the patient and their family. Collectively these tend to signal poor outcomes for those whose physical and mental health is already compromised.

It goes without saying that trust is crucially important in relationships between healthcare staff and the patients in their care. When caring for patients from different cultures, the establishment of trust is even more crucial so that those who have already been made vulnerable through illness are not set at greater disadvantage by being treated without consideration for their cultural needs. There is now an ample body of evidence to show that people who are unfamiliar with a healthcare system, especially those from immigrant communities, are far less inclined to make themselves heard – not because they might not have a sound cause, but because the prevailing institutional culture alienates rather than supports them.

The challenge to develop culturally sensitive services within healthcare invites the institution to engage both in attentive listening to these different voices and in collaborative creative thinking in order to see how the shape of services might be altered to accommodate different needs. The financial costs incurred in any modifications to service provision will be outweighed by the increase in mutual understanding and trust, which will have its own beneficial effect upon the patient population.

The routes to such changes lead through the educational pathways for all healthcare staff, as well as in careful attention to healthcare practice. This handbook will play its part well if, as a result of judiciously applying the information contained within it, staff gain an increased understanding of the different beliefs and practices contained within the various faith groups, and in so doing pay greater attention to the religious and cultural needs of those in their care. The groundswell of increased understanding and awareness that will be generated by this will in turn influence the pattern of service provision such that major discrepancies have a much stronger chance of being redressed.

References

1 America.gov. 15 August 2008: US minorities will be the majority by 2042, Census Bureau says; www.america.gov/st/diversity-english/2008/August 2008081514005xIrennef0.1078106.html (accessed 24 August 2008).

2 Kosmin BA, Mayer E and Keysar A. *American Religious Identification Survey*. New York: Graduate Center of the City University of New York; 2001, p. 9.

3 Trompenaars F. *Riding the Waves of Culture: understanding cultural diversity in business*. London: Nicholas Brealey; 1993.

4 Hofstede G. *Cultures and Organisations: software of the mind*. London: McGraw-Hill Book Company; 1991.

5 The United States Department of Health and Human Services, Office of Minority Health; www.omhrc (accessed 26 August 2008).

6 University of Minnesota, Center for Spirituality and Healing. *Cultural Competency Tools*; www.csh.umn.edu./modules/index.html (accessed July 27 2008).
   a Kleinman: Eight Questions
   b Berg: Cultural/Spiritual Assessment Tool
   c Berlin and Fowkes: LEARN Model
   d Levin, Like and Gottlieb: ETHNIC Framework.

Chapter 2

Spiritual care

What does it mean to be spiritual? What does it mean to be religious? In the previous chapter we have already noted the impact of increased ethnic diversity within Western Europe and the USA, and the loosening of the bonds between individuals and the ancient faith traditions and communities. The sociologist Thomas Luckmann, writing in the 1960s, offered a particularly insightful and prophetic comment about the shift in people's belief patterns: 'The modern sacred cosmos legitimates the retreat of the individual into the "private sphere" and sanctifies his (or her) subjective autonomy.'[1]

The shift and loosening of people's belief patterns and behaviours is likely to continue throughout the next decade and beyond, and it is perhaps too soon to speculate about the ultimate impact that these changes will have at every level of society. It is helpful to begin to understand this significant shift from a variety of perspectives, and not simply from the perspective of locating its cause solely within a secular and dominantly materialist culture. I believe that this shift marks a deeply significant change in how people believe, and what they need from and seek in any belief system. As western society has become characterised by highly individualist and more sophisticated behaviours and choices, this has manifested itself not only in an overt emphasis upon choice and personal development – whether in the shopping mall, the restaurant or the hospital – but also in relation to people's relationships at home, in the neighbourhood, and nationally. Given this broad context and emphasis, perhaps it is not surprising that individuals have taken another look at the faith of their parents and grandparents, and of the cultural community, and have begun to question their relationship to and with it in fundamental ways. Did the German theologian Dietrich Bonhoeffer have an inkling of this more open-weave context of individuality, society and religion in mind when he wrote of 'a world come of age'?[2] Although it might appear that Western society is becoming more secular, the reality may reflect a more private spirituality than an overt and communal religious practice. Again Thomas Luckmann seems to have the apposite term for this development – he calls it 'Invisible Religion.'[1]

It would seem that the challenge to religious institutions is to engage with these changes in ways that open and maintain a creative dialogue with those who question them and what they represent. Given this context, it becomes possible to recognise that many people may not necessarily have taken their leave of God and belief, but that they have detached themselves from the faith families. As a healthcare chaplain working in the UK National Health Service (NHS), I encounter many people – staff and patients – who no longer have an active adherent faith, but who do have an active spiritual life which draws upon one or more religions in positive ways to inform and enrich their lives. Equally, there are many people who describe themselves as spiritual without having any relationship to any specific faith tradition.

Believing without belonging has therefore become far more common-place among many more people. In the USA, the ARIS Survey 2001 asked respondents 'What is your religion, if any?' The replies indicated fluidity in the variety of adherence, identification and affiliation among the popula-tion. The authors of the Survey sought to capture this fluidity in the following terms: 'identification as a state of heart and mind and affiliation as a social condition.'[1]

However, even these terms will contain diverse and subjective mean-ings and interpretations as individuals attach different significance and value to each of them. The authors of the ARIS Survey also suggest that:

> *religious identification may well be a social marker as much as a marker designating a specific set of beliefs. For some it may be a reflection of a community or family anchor point to one's sense of self. For others still it may simply be the 'gut response' evoked by the question 'What is your religion, if any?', without any wider emotional, social or philosophical ramifications.*[1]

Given the increase in this exciting and perhaps rather puzzling diversity and fluidity in relation to religious belief, affiliation and identification within the populations of Western Europe and the USA, it is clear that, although religious belief may appear to be waning in terms of traditional practices of participating in a local faith community, its influence upon the way that people live their lives is not decreasing. What emerges is evidence that for many people it is possible to be culturally religious (e.g. many Jewish people have this relationship to their religion), while others may engage in non-religious spiritual practices as a means of investing their lives with meaning and purpose.

So what does it mean to be spiritual? And what is the place of religion within spiritual care as provided in healthcare institutions? Where does 'spiritual' belong? What is 'spiritual care'? There are further questions. Is any spirituality and spiritual discipline found only within and belonging to religion? Does religion have the sole and prior ownership of anything spiritual? Is it possible to have a spiritual life while not professing any religious adherence or specific faith? What difference, if any, is there between spirituality and religion?

This chapter will begin to map some of the routes that have been taken so far, and which might be taken, in response to some of these questions.

Yet both the questions and their answers belong rightly within the public as well as the private domain. Naturally they belong centrally within the domain of the main religions and of all who seek to engage with a spiritual life and to derive meaning and purpose for their lives through it.

A dictionary definition of the word 'spiritual' presents us first with a non-specific concept: 'of or relating to, or affecting the human spirit as opposed to material or physical things.'[3] Secondly, it offers us a more focused definition: 'of or relating to religion or religious belief.' A dictionary definition of religion provides several linked responses: 'the belief in and worship of a superhuman controlling power, especially a personal God or gods; a particular system of faith and worship; a pursuit or interest.'[4] A religion is a system of faith and worship, both of which express spirituality. Each religion has its own characteristics and, at best, provides room and encouragement for the exploration and expression of a variety of spiritualities within the overall framework of the beliefs, traditions and practices of the faith. It must be emphasised that religion and a religious belief should never exclude spirituality and a spiritual discipline or framework. Conversely, it should never be assumed that because a person does not subscribe to a particular religion they do not have any spirituality or interest in seeking spiritual meaning for their life.

Although such definitions provide us with a starting point, some might regard them as unhelpful and limiting. However, we can ask the following question: 'What affects our spirit?' We might begin to answer this question in terms of emotions as well as in terms of external factors that have a direct effect upon our lives, both practically and in relation to how we feel. We might also ask, in relation to this question, 'Who affects our spirit?' Our response to this question will begin to engage us in a consideration of the significant relationships that we have had and still have, and how these relationships nourish our spirit and our sense of purpose, of belonging, and of meaning in our lives.

When considering what it means to be spiritual, it is helpful to consider not only any particular religious belief that a person may have, but also other aspects of their life which they regard as important – not only their relationships, but also their work, hobbies, the sports they enjoy, etc. Some people take a distinctly philosophical and non-religious approach to life that excludes any reference to a power other than themselves. Examples of such an approach – which could be termed a belief system – include atheism, existentialism and humanism. However, whether approached from the context of religious faith or from the context of a specific or general philosophical and existential understanding, the search for meaning and purpose in life is common to all, and provides a foundation from which to begin to frame a broader set of definitions of what we understand the term 'spiritual' to mean, and how spiritual care within healthcare environments might be formulated.

So it may be misleading to think that because the number of people who profess any form of religious faith and practice would seem to be dwindling in western society, an interest in and curiosity about a spiritual element to human existence is also declining. There appears to be no such decline. By contrast, there is evidence of increased interest in New Age belief systems, as well as an eager market for what have been termed 'human potential movements.'[5] Those whose curiosity does not take them into such movements often retain or initiate a new connection with a traditional religion, while not wishing to subscribe entirely to its dogma and practices. Such people engage in what is known as 'supermarket religion' – taking elements from the shelves of several religions which have some meaning for them and which they can use as resources for their lives.

Another misleading understanding is that western society has become essentially materialistic and secular. Apart from the increase in the number of people who are actively seeking to discover more about different spiritual disciplines and traditions, with a view to engaging with one or more of them, there has been no significant decline in the number of people who adhere to common religion. Although a spiritual or religious belief and practice is regarded as a private matter, despite the emphasis upon supermarket religion, a belief is never entirely self-generated, but emerges not only in relation to the person's disposition in terms of thought and feeling, but also in relation to the prevailing context. Thus it may be more accurate to talk in terms of a common religion rather than of (and only exclusively of) a private one. Common religion encompasses the less mainstream elements of faith, belief and practice. Some aspects of common religion will have strong links with the orthodox beliefs of a particular religion, while others will be associated with different religious beliefs, or with practices dissociated from the belief system. Even within such a pattern there will be considerable variation in the beliefs, so that it becomes easier to think of these as being set within a very broad spectrum. This type of relationship with orthodox, mainstream religion is not restricted to the Christian tradition, but can be found within other religions, although to a lesser degree. This notion may tally with the ARIS reflection upon the difference between identification (common religion) and affiliation (a matter of active commitment and participation).

Common religion encompasses such habits as requesting a religious service from the local church (or Temple, Mosque, Synagogue, etc.) without the individual ever having had a strong connection with the faith community, except in some peripheral way. Within a healthcare setting, this request may be reformulated as requesting a Chaplain to attend a death or to officiate at an emergency baptism (if the patient is a Christian), or to arrange a wedding for a terminally ill patient. The provision of the rite does not depend upon the devotion and faith commitment of the person who makes the request. However nominal the person's attachment to the faith community (which the Chaplain represents at that point) might be, their strong spiritual and emotional need for the particular rite of passage to be provided at that time and in that particular circumstance overrides this.

Another category that has been proposed to try to encapsulate the pattern of believing but not belonging entirely is that of customary religion.[5] This term relates to a set of beliefs that still retains a connection, however loose, with the official teaching of the Roman Catholic Church. In a hospital setting, this is manifested as a request for the Catholic Chaplain to provide 'Last Rites' (a sacramental ministry of anointing with holy oil and administration of Holy Communion), even though the patient may have lapsed for many years and may even have turned away from the beliefs and practices of the faith. This represents one end of the broad spectrum of common or customary religion in which there are frequent strong links and associations with the Christian faith. At the other end of this spectrum may be found beliefs and practices that are now more closely linked with New Age practices. These include spiritual healing outside the remit of the Church's ministry of healing provided by registered Spiritual Healers, as well as the paranormal, and a further spectrum of psychic practices. These practices and the belief systems that they contain are not easily quantified or set within a clearly defined framework of belief (and it might be asked whether they need to be), but they are frequently a very forceful element of a person's response to crisis. For example, an acutely ill patient may be in bed surrounded by religious artefacts and charms belonging to several faiths, and to none in particular, even though their religion has been given as Hindu.

Many people are happy to admit that they 'believe' but that they no longer 'belong' to a particular faith community, as if they have grown out of it as well as away from it. This reflects the 'supermarket' approach to religion, and is reminiscent of the thought that 'one is nearer God's heart in a garden than anywhere else on earth.' This particular approach is relevant to an individual who does not make an active choice to pursue the 'Ariadne thread'[6] of curiosity, faith and belonging any further. The consequence may be that such individuals are left without a framework for further enquiry and development, and may tend to drift into other even more formless expressions and experiences of the religious and the spiritual. This pattern is in line with the postmodern emphasis upon fragmentation and self-fulfilment – that the individual will be able to construct from the fragments a coherent belief system for him- or herself.

By contrast with the free-flowing individual approach to belief and belonging, there is another pattern of modern religious behaviour that moves in the opposite direction, towards a reassertion of traditional beliefs. Conservatism within religion is very much alive and well, and accounts for much that is in protest against what appear to be permissive and highly individual cultural patterns. Yet such conservatism may also be found within secular cultures and competes with its religious counterparts. So even at the conservative end of this very broad and lengthy spectrum there is a bewildering variety of beliefs and practices that are in active use. Healthcare will benefit from an awareness of these nuances in order to avoid the easy stereotype and to be able to engage with the patient in their care.

Both within and without religious communities (faith families) there is a developing emphasis upon what could be termed 'right relationship' – with oneself, with others, with one's physical environment and with the global environment. This reflects an organic approach to life that regards everything as sacred and as being in relationship, so that if one part of the body is unhealthy, the entire body (the globe) suffers.

New Age movements place great emphasis upon these varied and related elements of right relationship, seeking and working towards wholeness. Wholeness then becomes a spiritual concept that emphasises the sacredness of all life. This belief is found among many ancient beliefs, such as the Native American traditions and many African tribal religions, as well as within the varied manifestations of Paganism. New Age spirituality is, in general, distanced from the major faiths and their teachings, although the common thread to each is the emphasis upon right relationship, albeit primarily with God, with all other relationships consequentially falling into rightness. New Age beliefs are often regarded, perhaps unhelpfully, as rivals of orthodox belief patterns, especially since there is no pressure with regard to individual assent to a particular dogma, which is often seen as a major advantage.

As increasing numbers of people turn to unconventional and untraditional spiritual pathways, so the 'marketplace' of religions is open to fresh influences which have the potential to assist in the reframing of old debates, tensions and sometimes rather proprietorial attitudes towards what is spiritual and what is religious into more expansive exploration.

Essentially there seems to be no place for any dichotomy between the practice of a religion and a spiritual life – together they represent the two sides of the same coin – although the quality of both will vary and will be dependent upon external factors such as the cultural environment, the size of the faith community, the freedom to observe one's religion, the personality of the person concerned and the various influences upon them, as well as upon their personal preferences for certain aspects of their faith. As the earlier parts of this chapter have illustrated, a spiritual life may take many forms and have different emphases. Some of these will overlap with concepts that are found in other areas, while others will belong only to a particular religion or spiritual movement.

It is important to emphasise that the main religions, as well as some of the newly emergent spiritual movements, have tremendous resources for the creation, nourishing and sustaining of a spiritual life – taproots reaching into deep wells whose foundations were set thousands of years ago. Yet it is also possible to say that spirituality, and a spiritual life, are not necessarily the preserve of the main religions or indeed of any spiritual development movement. It seems reasonable to assert that the search for a meaning and purpose for our human existence is common to us all, and is not only the domain of those who have a religious faith. The form that this search takes is necessarily and significantly varied. It also seems reasonable to assert that there are likely to be areas of commonality where the religious and the philosophical, alongside other approaches to living one's life, have shared sets of meaning. Shared sets of meaning would include such things as the importance of relationship (with oneself, with others, and with the past, the present and the future), the importance and significance of place, the importance of belonging and of contributing and giving to and receiving from others, and the significance and meaning of loss in all its forms.

It is possible to regard spirituality as being akin to a kaleidoscope encompassing religious belief and practice, New Age movements and highly individual belief systems independent of any particular religious belief and dogma – the colours and patterns of each shifting and tumbling together and forming new patterns from former patterns. There is a developing research base with regard to spirituality, with particular reference to the spirituality of those who are ill. I have extrapolated some of the key elements which characterise spirituality, and in Boxes 2.1 and 2.2 I have set these alongside what I consider to be the key elements of a religious belief system.[7] It comes as no surprise to find that there are many elements common to both!

Disintegration – falling to pieces – is a common reaction to a life crisis, whether this takes place at the point of impact or whether it is delayed for an unspecified length of time. Many people 'hold themselves together' at the time of crisis, and later, when the immediate crisis is over, they allow themselves to 'fall apart' to some degree. In crisis our response is often that of 'fight or flight', when the adrenalin rush sometimes makes it difficult to respond rationally. One of the purposes of spiritual care, whether at a time of crisis or over a much longer period of time, is to facilitate the individual's response and to support them in articulating their deeper thoughts, feelings and needs. This can be summed up as a search for re-integration, or even simply integration – to seek for and find purpose and meaning in circumstances that feel devoid of all meaning. Whether or not this integrative work takes place within the framework of a particular religion will depend upon the person, but the context for all of the different approaches is that of a spiritual search and expression which allows for a richly varied set of responses from one or more elements that characterise spirituality.

A word of caution might be timely at this point. Throughout any developmental process that involves cultivating and sustaining a more thoroughly comprehensive understanding of spirituality and spiritual care, it is important to avoid creating overarching systems which attempt

Box 2.1: Attributes of spirituality

Meaning
The ontological significance of life; making sense of life situations; deriving purpose in existence.

Belief
Non-religious patterns and framework of belief; may or may not be influenced by some of the mainstream faiths and/or New Age beliefs.

Belonging
Relationships with those who share the same or similar beliefs; exploring these beliefs together; creating and experiencing community; sense of continuity.

Nurturing, sustaining
Rituals, prayers, symbols, special and meaningful activities that nourish one's inner life and maintain connectedness with others, with God or the divine, or with self at a deep level.

Value
Beliefs and standards that are cherished; concerning truth, beauty and worth of a thought, object or behaviour; often discussed as 'ultimate values.'

Transcendence
Experience and appreciation of a dimension beyond the self; expanding self-boundaries; sense of awareness of the Divine/God or a higher power.

Connecting
Relationship with self, others, God or a higher power, and the environment.

Becoming
An unfolding of life that demands reflection and experience; includes a sense of who one is and how one knows; a sense of life beyond death and continuing development.

Principles
Values, ethics and moral tenets to frame and influence one's thoughts, feelings, aspirations and behaviour towards others and self.

Reproduced from Hollins S (2005) Spirituality and religion: exploring the relationship. *Nursing Management* 12(6): 25–26. With permission from RCN Publishing Company.

Box 2.2: Attributes of religion

Meaning
Divine and ontological purpose, and significance of life; developing purpose; purpose through suffering.

Belief
Pattern and framework for one's life that can be challenged and challenging; sustaining, informing; guiding in relation to life crises; sanctity and purpose of life.

Belonging
The family of the faith; a sense of history and of future – both one's own and that of the faith community; sense of continuity.

Nurturing, sustaining
Prayers, worship, symbolism of language and ritual; seasons of the religious year; festivals; relationships arising from and nurtured within the faith community.

Transcendence
Seeking for and being found by God or the divine; going beyond self; relationship with God or the divine; life beyond the limitations of one's body, and immediate circumstances, beyond death.

Becoming
Growing in relationship to God or the divine; a sense of divine 'call' or invitation; response to this invitation.

Principles
Ethical and moral principles; framework for thought and behaviour related to truth, love, justice and compassion.

Connectedness
Relationship to others; relationship with local community and environment; service to others in the name of God or the divine.

Forgiveness, hope, love, joy and compassion
Divine attributes that are sought for one's life and that are exercised in relation to others and self.

Reproduced from Hollins S (2005) Spirituality and religion: exploring the relationship. *Nursing Management* 12(6): 25–26. With permission from RCN Publishing Company.

to apply a universal solution to the questions posed by both a religious and a religion-less spirituality. Allowance is best made for variation of expression.

Each of the main religions has a different concept of what it means to be spiritual – that is, to have a spiritual life or spirituality. This is in contrast with emerging constructs for spirituality, which tend to oversimplify. In the USA, the work of Larry and Laura Fahlberg and of Pamela Reed exemplifies such approaches. These approaches are not always relevant to people who belong to the major faiths who have very different understandings of what spiritual care means, and for whom the concept of pastoral care may be unusual. This emerging but overarching definition of spiritual care is closest to but not wholly aligned with Christian models. There are three main elements to this concept of spiritual care. The first is an emphasis upon holistic care, which considers the individual's feelings and any beliefs or philosophical framework for living. The second element emphasises the search for and discovery of meaning that can be articulated through beliefs and values. The third element emphasises a 'capacity for self-transcendence that is expressed by expanding personal boundaries intrapersonally, interpersonally and transpersonally – inward, outward and upward. Transcendence can be found within or beyond the self, depending upon one's religious or philosophical beliefs.'[8]

Ian Markham asserts that this definition of spirituality is merely a secular version of the Christian understanding of spirituality.[9] Such a definition is, according to Markham, reductionist in its approach, watering down the essential elements of orthodox concepts of spirituality from within Christianity alone. Although such reduced concepts of spirituality might be understood, if not accepted, by the Christian traditions, they are certainly more likely to be unacceptable to other major faiths, on the basis that these have a very different understanding of what spirituality is.

The concept of transcendence is alien to most of the major faiths. The spirituality of Islam emphasises the extinction of the self in Allah. This is not to be regarded negatively, but revered, for the purpose of the self is for it to merge with God. By contrast, Judaism emphasises the discovery of that which is spiritual in everyday life. This to some extent explains the food laws and other disciplines that practising Jewish people exercise, for these are reminders of the presence of God and of the 'transcendent significance'[10] of the normal and everyday. Hinduism does not really have a concept of transcendence. It emphasises that the divine is within each person. The task of each person is to make an inward journey and in so doing to encounter the divine – the cosmic self (Brahman). The Buddhist emphasis, by way of further contrast, is on the transience of all things and on ethical (right) living: 'Spirituality, then, is the cultivation of certain dispositions that integrate this awareness of the transient nature of all things into one's life.'[11]

There is an understandable reserve within the faith communities about the apparent ease with which any definition of spirituality can be developed for use within healthcare contexts. Each religion naturally exercises a different understanding of spirituality and its expression, so how can such diversity be encapsulated within one or two sentences? Another justifiable concern is that since spirituality is at the heart of the faiths, it is important first for this to be acknowledged and understood by healthcare providers, and for there to be encouragement to include a fuller understanding of the different religions and cultures within all training programmes. A bold yet creative move might be to engage members of the different religious groups in dialogue about what is meant by spirituality and spiritual care in the healthcare environment. One element of this dialogue could be to explore whether spirituality can be identified and developed apart from any religion, and if so, what the characteristics might be. My earlier reflections indicate that it is possible to discern an initial framework for understanding spirituality apart from a religious framework by considering existential themes, such as a search for meaning and belonging, or the importance and meaning of different kinds of relationship. Currently there are religious definitions of spirituality and there are also secular as well as philosophical definitions, but each operates within separate areas. The Christian traditions have developed and provided leadership within healthcare chaplaincy alongside their Jewish colleagues for many years. Representatives from the other major faiths are now joining them in this work. Alongside a developing understanding of spiritual care from within the faith traditions, the nursing communities have also provided an excellent seedbed for some secular and philosophical concepts of spirituality and spiritual care.

In any serious consideration of both cultural diversity and spiritual care within healthcare, it becomes clear that we have embarked upon the reclamation of the individual – a creative recognition of the person who is at the heart of any treatment. This recognition naturally leads to further reflection upon what it means to be a person. It also leads to the posing of searching questions concerned with religion and spirituality and how these inform and influence the person for whom we have a professional responsibility.

Some regard religion as being damaging to health (and there is strong evidence to support this view, just as there is strong evidence to support its beneficial influence upon health). Nevertheless, the vast knowledge and experience that the main religions possess both individually and collectively in relation to concepts of 'right living' (a balanced life) as well as in relation to the care of the sick and the dying must not be set aside as irrelevant to the age in which we live.

In this chapter I have only begun to outline some of the elements that can be found in any consideration of a spiritual life, what it means to be religious, and what it means to nourish spirituality, as well as considering how the divisions between what is regarded as secular and sacred are shifting. Within the overall context of cultural diversity the time has come to address these other crucial elements of diversity that reflect and give clues about what it means to be a person. These clues can no longer be reduced or disregarded by healthcare institutions as being peripheral to the well-being of patients.

References

1 Kosmin BA, Mayer E and Keysar A. *American Religious Identification Survey*. New York: Graduate Center of the City University of New York; 2001. pp. 14, 16.
2 Bonhoeffer D. *Letters and Papers from Prison*. London: Fontana Books; 1963. p. 118.
3 America.gov. 19 August 2008: The demographics of faith; www.America.gov/st/diversity-english/2008/August/20080819121858cmretrop0.5130633.html (accessed 24 August 2008).
4 America.gov. 15 August 2008: US minorities will be the majority by 2042, Census Bureau says; www.america.gov/st/diversity-english/2008/August 2008081514005xIrennef0.1078106.html (accessed 24 August 2008).
5 Pearsall J, editor. *The Concise Oxford English Dictionary*, revised 10th ed. Oxford: BCA by arrangement with Oxford University Press; 2001.
6 Davie G. Faith and belief: a sociological perspective. In: Cobb M and Robshaw V (eds) *The Spiritual Challenge of Healthcare*. Edinburgh: Elsevier; 1998, p. 92.
7 Hollins S. Keeping the faith. *Nurse Management*. 2005; 12: 25–6.
8 Hornsby-Smith M. *Roman Catholic Beliefs in England*. Cambridge: Cambridge University Press; 1991.
9 Markham I. Spirituality and world faiths. In: Cobb M and Robshaw V (eds) *The Spiritual Challenge of Healthcare*. Edinburgh: Elsevier; 1998, p. 77.
10 Hammarskjöld D (trans. Auden WH, Sjoberg L). *Markings*. London: Faber and Faber; 1964, p. 169.
11 Reed P. The enchantment of healthcare: a paradigm of spirituality. In: Cobb M and Robshaw V (eds) *The Spiritual Challenge of Healthcare*. Edinburgh: Elsevier; 1998, p. 42.

Chapter 3

Elements of care

For ease of reference, each section in Chapter 4 has a similar layout relating to the following areas. Where certain information has not been gathered the section is omitted.

- background and beliefs
- naming system
- religious obligations
- diet
- dress
- language
- birth
- personal hygiene
- gender, privacy and dignity
- attitude to illness
- blood transfusions
- contraception
- fertility treatment
- stem cell research where this information is known
- pastoral care
- dying and death
- autopsy
- organ and tissue donation

Chapter 4

Religions and other faith groups

- Baha'i
- Buddhist
- Christian including: Catholic, Friends (Quakers), Greek Orthodox, Russian Orthodox, Seventh Day Adventists
- Other groups
  - Christian Science
  - Jehovah's Witness
  - Mormon (Church of Jesus Christ of Latter-Day Saints)
  - Rastafari
- Hindu
- Muslim
- American Indian/Alaska Natives
- Jain
- Jewish
- Pagan including: Wiccan, Heathenry
- Sikh
- Zoroastrian
- **Appendix:**
  - Care of the Chinese patient
  - Care of the Latino patient
  - Care of the Somali patient
  - Care of the Vietnamese patient

Baha'i

Background and beliefs

- The Baha'i faith was founded in Persia in 1844 by Husayn Ali, known to Baha'is as Baha'u'llah (Glory of God). It was declared as a new religion, different to Shia Islam practised in Iran.
- Three of the 12 key beliefs are as follows:
  - belief in one God (oneness of God)
  - the unity of mankind (oneness of humankind)
  - the common foundation of all religions (oneness of Religion).
- Unity is a central theme of the Baha'i faith. Baha'is believe that there has only ever been one religion and one God, although people have called him by different names. Baha'is believe that Baha'u'llah was the great messenger who would bring peace to the world.
- Baha'is have a great respect for life. Each person has a soul that comes into being at conception. During a person's lifetime, the soul acquires spiritual attributes required for the next stage of existence, which occurs at death.
- The Baha'i faith is an independent world religion with its own laws and ordinances.
- Baha'is have a great respect for doctors and are encouraged to consult the best possible medical advice when ill.

Naming system

The manner of addressing the person will be influenced by their ethnic origin.

Religious obligations

There are three obligatory daily prayers, of which one must be said. Baha'is turn in the direction of Bahji in Israel – the burial place of Baha'u'llah.

Diet

- There are no dietary restrictions. Some Baha'is may be vegetarian, but this is not a religious requirement. Habit-forming drugs are forbidden.
- Fasting takes place each year during the holy season from 2 to 20 March. This is a time of spiritual regeneration. From sunrise to sunset each day Baha'is fast. During sickness, pregnancy and menstruation the

fast is lifted. Mothers who are breastfeeding, and people under 15 years or over 70 years of age are exempted from fasting.

Dress

In general there are no religious obligations with regard to everyday wear.

Language

Baha'i is an ethnically diverse religion. Baha'i families may speak several languages other than English, depending on their cultural background.

Birth

The birth of a child is a time of joy. There are no rituals associated with birth.

Personal hygiene

Baha'is require no special conditions with regard to washing, bathing, etc. Some may wish to wash before their daily prayer.

Gender, privacy and dignity

Baha'is do not object to being examined by doctors of the opposite sex.

Attitude to illness

Baha'is have great respect for scientifically-based medical opinion, and they are encouraged to seek out and comply with the best advice. Alongside medication the Baha'is also strongly believe in the power of prayer in the healing process. They are also open to natural and lifestyle choices that support healing.

Blood transfusions

Baha'is have no objection to blood transfusions.

Contraception

Family planning is left to the personal conscience of the Baha'i, but the following considerations should be borne in mind.

- Sterilisation in either sex is strongly discouraged. In cases where a medical condition is relevant to the decision, the individual should seek qualified advice.
- Methods of contraception that prevent implantation of the fertilised ovum are unacceptable, as Baha'is believe that the soul comes into being at conception.

Fertility treatment

Baha'is will make decisions relating to fertility treatment on an individual basis, with the underlying commitment to the sustaining of life.

Stem cell research

As Baha'is believe in harmony between science and religion they are likely to maintain an open regard for this research.

Pastoral care

Baha'is will welcome visits by members of their local Spiritual Assembly.

Dying and death

- The body of a person is believed to be a vehicle of the soul, so Baha'is treat the body of a deceased person with great respect.
- Funeral laws prohibit embalming
- The relatives or friends of Baha'is will wish to say prayers for the dead.
- Baha'i law prescribes that burial should take place at a distance of not more than one hour's journey from the place of death.
- Funerals are normally arranged by the family of the deceased if available, or on occasion by the Spiritual Assembly.

Autopsy

There are no objections to autopsies.

Organ and tissue donation

- Baha'is may leave their bodies for scientific research.
- Baha'is may donate organs and/or tissue for transplantation.

Buddhist

Background and beliefs

- This is the way of life for the people who follow the teachings of Buddha. The faith focuses on Mahatma Gautam Shakyamuni Buddha, who lived in India over 2500 years ago. He is worshipped not as a god, but as the founder of a way of life. Buddha is believed to have found the middle way between luxuries and asceticism. This is called the Eightfold Path to enlightenment, which is symbolised by an eight-spoked wheel.
- Buddhism is a highly individual spiritual path, as the religion has no single creed, authority or sacred book.
- Buddhism exists in a variety of forms, adapting itself to the cultures and peoples that engage in it.
- One of Buddhism's central pillars is the practice of The Four Immeasurable Minds:
  - love
  - compassion
  - joy
  - equanimity or non-attachment.
- Buddhists regard the mind and body as a single unit.
- Buddhism does not have a belief system. Its emphasis is upon teachings used as guides in daily life. The Five Precepts are the basic rules for daily living for lay Buddhists:
  - nonharming
  - nonstealing
  - sexual responsibility
  - mindful speech
  - drink or drugs which could cloud the mind
- Buddhists find support in the Buddha, in his teachings and in the community of Buddhists. They strive to live skilfully – that is, following the Buddhist precepts and teachings, being mindful of the effect of their behaviour upon others, and leading a peaceful existence that values humility. Ethical thinking and right actions are also important.
- Central to the Buddhist belief is the injunction not to cause harm to others, and to help all beings.
- The Buddhist aim is to achieve Nirvana – that is, a state of liberation characterised by freedom from suffering, death and rebirth.
- Buddhists believe in rebirth (not reincarnation), and believe that their actions in this life will affect the quality of the next. Therefore they accept all responsibility for their actions.

Naming system

- It is usual for Buddhists to have two or more names, the first of which may be the family name, and the second or subsequent name(s) the given name(s).
- It is advisable to ask first for the family name, and to use this as the surname.

Language

Buddhist families may speak several languages other than English, including Chinese, Lao, Thai and Vietnamese.

Religious obligations

- Buddhist religious practice is very variable, depending upon the individual. It may include chanting and meditation.
- A peaceful environment is generally helpful.
- An image of the Buddha may be a good support to patients.
- Prayer beads may also be helpful.

Diet

- Diet varies according to the climate of the country. Generally speaking, Buddhists are vegetarian, as the notion of non-harm is central to Buddhist teaching.
- Salt-free salads, rice, vegetables and fruit are generally acceptable foods.
- Ordained and strict Buddhists may be vegan and may choose not to eat after midday. A modest diet signifies awareness that people generally eat more than they need.
- Fasting is neither a feature nor a practice among most Buddhists, with the exception of monks and nuns. Most fasting takes place on New Moon and Full Moon days, but there are also other festival days (e.g. Buddha's birthday, his death day, his enlightenment, his first sermon, and others).

Dress

- Generally there are no religious requirements concerning forms of everyday dress for lay Buddhists.
- Ordained monks and nuns are distinguished by their brightly coloured robes.

Birth

- A peaceful birth environment will be appreciated.
- No special ceremonies are required. A blessing may be performed later.

Personal hygiene

- There are no special obligations, but the following may be required:
  - a container of water for washing if the toilet is separate from the bathroom
  - showers are preferable to baths.
- Buddhists from different parts of the world may follow various social customs.

Gender, privacy and dignity

- There are no special obligations.
- Buddhist monks or nuns will prefer to be treated by a member of staff of the same sex. They may also have specific needs related to their vows.

Attitude to illness

- Helping people is fundamental to Buddhist ideas, so Buddhists will respect the medical staff for their help.
- Illness and suffering will be understood in relation to the Four Noble Truths:
  - the truth of suffering
  - the truth of the cause of suffering
  - the truth of the cessation of suffering
  - the Eightfold Path.
- Buddhists may prefer to maintain a clear mind when terminally ill. This may involve the refusal of pain-relieving drugs if these would impair mental alertness.
- Buddhists may traditionally and culturally favour the use of home remedies.

Blood transfusions

- There are no religious objections to blood transfusions.
- Buddhists generally regard the donation of blood an excellent means of giving to someone else.

Contraception

- This is not a cause of concern to Buddhists, who would usually practise any of the conventional methods.
- Any method of contraception that is used should be one which safeguards the normal development of the baby if conceived
- Most Buddhists would not consent to an abortion because it would compromise the sanctity of all living beings.

Fertility treatment

The Five Precepts (and other beliefs) will provide the framework for all decisions relating to fertility treatment. Therefore it is important to attend to the individual's approach in the light of these beliefs.

Stem cell research

- Buddhist scholars and communities are divided on this subject.
- There are two contrasting Buddhist beliefs in this matter:
    - that one should do no harm to a living being
    - the pursuit of knowledge.
- Some scholars agree that stem cell research is in accordance with the Buddhist tenet of seeking knowledge and ending human suffering.
- Other scholars say that stem cell research violates the concept of not harming a living being.

Pastoral care

- Buddhist patients may welcome visits by other members of the local Buddhist community.
- Patients may require the help of a chaplain in arranging a time at which meditation may take place.

Dying and death

- Most Buddhists will provide medical staff with the name of the person to contact in the event of their death if this differs from their next of kin/named person.
- The death of a person is viewed as a very important time. The body should be treated with the greatest care and respect, and it should be disturbed only for special reasons and with appropriate care.
- Buddhists regard the preparation for death as crucially important. This overrides any rituals associated with death.

- There is no single Buddhist ritual before, at the time of or after death. Examples of some practices are listed below.
  - A Buddhist priest or monk of the same school of Buddhism could be informed immediately so that prayers may be recited as soon as possible after the death.
  - Relatives/friends may wish the body to remain where it is until a priest is able to attend.
  - Sufficient time will be required for the prayers to be said.
  - It may not always be necessary for the priest to be present to recite prayers that may be recited at a distance (e.g. in a temple).
  - In some traditions it is customary for the body to remain at the place of death for up to 7 days to allow rebirth to take place. However, it is unusual for this practice to be enforced by relatives within a healthcare setting, although healthcare staff need to be aware of this practice.
- Buddhists generally prefer cremation to burial, as it is a symbol of the impermanence of the body.

Autopsy

There are no objections to autopsies.

Organ and tissue donation

- In Buddhism there are no injunctions for or against organ donation. Central to Buddhism is a wish to relieve suffering, and there may be circumstances in which organ donation may be seen as an act of charity.
- Each decision will depend upon the feelings of those involved and the teachings of the different schools of Buddhism.

Christian

Background and beliefs

Christianity begins with the person of Jesus Christ who lived over 2000 years ago, and whom Christians believe to be both human and divine. Christians understand God to be one being, but revealed in three distinct 'persons': Father, Son and Holy Spirit. Christians believe that God revealed himself in the life, death and the resurrection of Jesus Christ.

Christians believe that God's forgiveness and healing extend to all people through the self-giving (sacrifice) of Jesus Christ on the cross. They believe that through the death of Christ death itself has been overcome and that eternal life, which spans both earthly and spiritual worlds, is a gift of God to all in and through Christ.

The Church is the community of the believers whose worship and service of god in the world extends his kingdom of love, truth, justice and peace. Christians believe in living according to the loving nature of God as revealed in Jesus' life and death, helped in this by the Holy Spirit, and by communicating with God through prayer.

Sunday is the usual day on which Christians gather together for worship as it is believed to be the day of the week on which Jesus was raised from the dead, bringing to birth a new order or relationship with God.

There is immense diversity of belief, worship, and service within the many different denominations of the Christian faith, with a variety of cultural and ethnic influences adding to its richness.

General guidance

This information is for guidance only. It does not provide comprehensive information for each of the Christian traditions and denominations within them. For further, detailed, information for each of the denominations the Resources section provides signposts to assist your journey of exploration. Some specific detail is provided for particular denominations later in this section. The breadth of belief, tradition and practice within and between denominations serves to emphasise the requirement to be led by the needs of the Christian patient at all times in matters of personal faith and spiritual care.

Naming system

- The term 'Christian name' refers to the first name that a person is given at their baptism. Historically someone who became a Christian during adulthood would receive a new 'baptismal' name to signify their new

life in Christ. This name would often be the name of a Biblical character or a saint.
- A Christian name now generally refers to the forename of a person which is followed by the family name.

Religious obligations

- Advent, Christmas, Ash Wednesday, Lent, Easter, Ascension Day, and Pentecost are the major holy seasons of the church's year, when attendance at worship is expected.
- There is a rich diversity of worship traditions within the Church as a whole and between different denominations, e.g. Orthodox Christians keep the festivals of Christmas and Easter on dates different to those kept by mainline Protestant and Catholic Christians.
- Prayer is very important for Christians who are encouraged to develop their own pattern and discipline that includes private prayer alongside attending worship at church.
- Christian patients may:
  - wish for privacy in order to maintain their own private prayer
  - welcome the opportunity to receive the sacrament of Holy Communion not only at times of particular stress (i.e. before surgery) but on a regular basis while hospitalised
  - welcome the opportunity to receive anointing and laying on of hands for healing.

Diet

- Generally Christians are not forbidden to eat any particular kinds of food or to abstain from alcohol.
- Some Christian denominations ban the consumption of stimulating drinks altogether and support vegetarianism.
- Ash Wednesday, marking the beginning of a holy season of penitence and renewal, is a day of fasting. How much an individual fasts is left up to their own discipline and other needs (e.g. medical, pregnancy etc).
- Some Christians maintain a strict adherence to a Lenten discipline throughout the 6 week period up to Easter by not eating more luxurious kinds of food.
- Some Christians may wish to fast before receiving Holy Communion (especially in the early morning).

Dress

- In general Christians are not obliged to dress in a particular way in terms of everyday wear.

- Some denominations may apply a dress code (e.g. Amish, Conservative Quakers).
- Monks or nuns (religious) may have clothes which would include the wearing of robes and a head-covering (for women).

Language

Christianity is ethnically diverse and members of Christian families may speak several languages other than English

Birth

- For many Christians it is important for a baby to be baptised (christened).
- Many Christian traditions practise 'Believers' Baptism' only for individuals old enough to speak for themselves. Infants are brought to church for a blessing (e.g. a thanksgiving for the birth of a child).
- If a baby is near to death an emergency baptism may be performed by the Healthcare Chaplain or by the family's local minister, or by a nurse in the absence of an ordained cleric.
- The baptism of a dead baby is not normal practice.
- A service of blessing (or blessing and naming) may be offered at the time of death or within a reasonable period afterwards.

Personal hygiene

There are no special religious obligations with regard to hygiene.

Gender, privacy and dignity

In general there are no special religious obligations. However, there may be variations within and between denominations so it is best to be led by the patient.

Attitude to illness

- Christian teaching encourages the faithful to respond to their illness as positively as possible, entrusting themselves to God's healing care.
- Christian teaching also undergirds a recognition of the place of suffering within human experience and what we may learn from this.

Blood transfusions

There are no religious restrictions upon blood transfusions.

Contraception

- In general Christians make decisions regarding contraception privately, sometimes after consultation with their Priest/Minister.
- The official statement of the Catholic Church is that contraception is not permitted. Many Catholic couples make their own autonomous decision in this respect.

Fertility treatment

There are no major religious grounds against fertility treatment as it would be consistent with theological principles. However, individual Christian traditions may have particular religious guidance about fertility treatment.

Stem cell research

Not all denominations have provided a formal statement on this issue. Some denominations may choose not to make a formal statement.

Pastoral care

- Christian patients may welcome supportive visits from members of their local church as well as from the Healthcare Chaplain.
- Pastoral care may include prayers, readings from Scripture and emotional and spiritual support in response to the needs of the patient.
- Patients welcome privacy when being visited by a Chaplain or by a Priest/Minister of their own church

Dying and death

- Terminally ill patients may welcome the chance to prepare themselves for death by means of prayers with family, friends and their local Priest/ Minister and/or the Healthcare Chaplain.
- Anticipation of the patient's needs as they approach death will be welcomed.
- The patient and/or their relatives may ask for a Chaplain or their own Priest/Minister to visit.
- After the patient has died the Chaplain, local Priest or Minister may still attend to say prayers, and to support the relatives.

Autopsy

Generally there are no religious objections to autopsies.

Organ and tissue donation

- Enabling life to be lived as fully as possible is consistent with the teachings of Jesus Christ.
- Christians are encouraged to help others in need, so discussing organ donation with the patient's family may be appropriate.

Catholic

- Catholic teaching encourages the participation of the church at all stages of illness.
- Catholic patients may welcome all or some of the various kinds of religious, pastoral and spiritual support that can be provided by their own local Priest and/or by the Catholic chaplain in the hospital.
- Patients and their relatives welcome the opportunity to attend Mass in the hospital chapel if this is provided, or for the Sacrament to be brought to the patient at the bedside.
- Patients may wish to make their confession to a Priest.
- Patients may wish to celebrate the Sacrament of the Sick especially at times of crisis or in advance of major surgery.

Dying and death

- Patients may wish their Priest and/or the Catholic chaplain to recite Prayers for the Dying.
- Prayers for the Dead will be said after the patient has died.

Organ and tissue donation

There are no religious objections to this

Stem cell research

The Conference of Catholic Bishops supports adult stem cell research but opposes embryonic stem cell research since it creates or destroys human embryos

Friends (Quakers)

The Religious Society of Friends (Quakers) originated in mid-seventeenth century England. Its core assumption is that each individual has the capacity for direct communion with the Divine, unmediated by ritual, clergy or scripture. Friends meet for worship in silence, and 'wait expectantly' for divine visitation, unguided by formal clergy. Individuals may offer messages during worship, if so inspired, but there is no pre-planned ministry or other service. Although the tradition is Christian today some liberal Quakers do not consider themselves to be Christian, but rather to be Universalists. There is no Quaker Creed (Statement of Faith) but Friends are expected to seek guidance from the Inward Light in their personal interpretations of traditional testimonies.

Basic precepts

- That all people are sacred, potential ministers of God's word.
- All people have capacity for direct unmediated revelation from God.
- Guidance from such revelation is valued above all other teachings although the interpretation of it is not inerrant and must be tested in a variety of ways.
- God's revelation is continuing and new truths may be revealed.
- Individuals are expected to seek God's guidance individually and as a community in the conduct of their lives.
- Quakers do not take oaths. They will affirm rather than swear.
- Religious holidays have not been celebrated although Christmas and Easter have now been adopted as cultural practice.
- Traditionally, Quakers have valued and been guided by the principles of:
  - peace (including pacifism with respect to war and capital punishment)
  - simplicity
  - equality, integrity, community
  - environmental stewardship. Individual interpretations of how to apply these principles varies from person to person. For example, a cancer patient may choose a treatment that will not produce toxic waste (environmental stewardship); another individual might choose a generic medication, even when their health insurance covers a more expensive drug (simplicity).

Diet

Many Friends are vegetarian.

Birth, stillbirth and miscarriage

Individuals are free to respond in their own ways.

Pastoral care

- Patients may appreciate periods of silence for worship.
- A worship or 'clearness committee' (a group that provides spiritual and practical help in decision-making) from the Meeting. These informal groups may be as important to the person as Ordained Clergy are to other denominations.
- Time: Quakers make decisions slowly. In a group they wait for unity rather than voting. At times of crisis they will prefer to wait and expect to receive spiritual guidance.
- Caregivers may welcome the opportunity to use a discrete space where they can worship with or on behalf of a patient (e.g. before/during surgery).

Dying and death

- There are no particular traditions or rituals. During the final days members of the Community will visit the dying person to participate in the experience of life's completion.
- Many Friends choose cremation.

Organ and tissue donation

Donation is not uncommon amongst Friends

Greek Orthodox

- Members of the Greek Orthodox Church would expect pastoral and spiritual support as set out in the previous section from their own Priest, and only from the Hospital Chaplain if he is of the same tradition.
- Specifically they would welcome prayers for healing, Holy Communion, Anointing with Holy Unction for healing of soul and body.
- Parishioners are expected to notify their Priest if they go into hospital.

Dying and death

The Orthodox Church insists that the body be buried

Autopsy

- An autopsy may be performed in accordance with the law, with the permission of the next of kin.
- The Orthodox Church expects that the body of the deceased be treated with respect and dignity.

Organ and tissue donation

- The donation of an organ from a deceased person is an act of love that helps to make possible a longer fuller life for the recipient.
- These donations are acceptable if the deceased donor has willed this or if surviving relatives permit it providing this is in harmony with the desires of the deceased.
- Organ transplants should never be commercialised nor take place without proper consent, nor put in jeopardy the identity of the donor or recipient.
- The death of the donor should not be hastened in order to harvest organs for transplantation to another person.

Russian Orthodox

- It is customary for the families of Orthodox Christians whether of Russian or any ancestry to inform their parish priests of hospitalisation.
- Orthodox Christians should not be offered the Sacraments from non-Orthodox Christian clergy as the Church does not permit intercommunion.
- If the family has not contacted the parish priest the hospital chaplaincy staff should contact a priest.

Fertility treatment, organ and tissue donation, autopsy

The Church has specific guidelines on these matters but these are generally communicated by the parish priest who works with the family.

Seventh Day Adventists

- Seventh Day Adventists are Christians in the Protestant Tradition. They maintain a Saturday Sabbath tradition.
- Members have a strong sense of family and community life.
- Members of this Church are forbidden to smoke, drink alcohol or use any other intoxicating substance.
- Some members may be vegetarian.
- Whenever Adventists choose to leave the Church it is recognised that they are not only leaving a church but also a culture. This may cause considerable distress to those concerned.
- Patients will welcome the pastoral and spiritual support of their local Pastor and other representatives of the SDA community.

Dying and death

Burial is preferred to cremation.

Organ and tissue donation

There may be objections to this on religious grounds.

Autopsy

There may be objections to autopsies on religious grounds.

Acknowledgements

Friends: Quaker Information Center (USA and London UK) Chel Avery and Simon Best, Directors, respectively.

Greek Orthodox: Father James Kordaris, Director Outreach and Evangelism, Greek Orthodox Church USA.

Health Care Chaplains: Rev'd Jenny Lannom, Manager Pastoral Education, Chaplaincy Services, Presbyterian Healthcare Services, Albuquerque, New Mexico.

Russian Orthodox Church: Father John Matusiak, OCA Web Team, Russian Orthodox Church.

Other groups

Christian Science

Background and beliefs

Christian Science, established by Mary Baker Eddy, is a system of understanding and applying spiritual ideas to all aspects of life, including the healing or cure of disease. Christian Science is fully explained in Eddy's primary work, *Science and Health with Key to the Scriptures*. This healing system has been practised around the world for over a century by individuals of various faith traditions, as well as by those with no formal faith tradition. Some individuals choose to become members of the Church of Christ, Scientist, a church established by Mary Baker Eddy to make Christian Science healing more widely known and accessible.

Central to the practice of Christian Science is respect for individual choice in matters of healthcare or any other aspect of daily life. Many Christian Scientists rely on prayer for healing of diseases and disorders. However, individuals are free to choose conventional medical treatment.

Christian Science is based on the life, teaching and work of Jesus Christ.

- Christian Scientists do not have a common creed.
- Lay Christian Science practitioners are trained in Church principles and present a prayer-based healing ministry to members and to the public as an alternative to conventional medical treatment.
- The Church interprets and uses the traditional Sacraments of the mainstream Christian denominations differently: Baptism is regarded as the continual purification of thought and deed; The Eucharist is regarded as *spiritual communion with the one God, which is celebrated with silent prayer and Christian living*.
- Christian Scientists do not have an antagonistic approach to traditional medical practitioners. They simply prefer to choose prayer as treatment for themselves and their children on the basis of past experience of the efficacy of prayer.
- The regeneration of heart and mind that accompanies physical healing is often the most significant for individuals.
- The teachings of Jesus Christ are central to Christian Science.
- Christian Scientists believe that healing is not accomplished through blind faith but through a deepening understanding of God and an acceptance that humans are made in God's image and likeness.
- Christian Scientists pray for themselves, but may also call upon the support of a practitioner: men and women who offer their services of prayer on a voluntary basis. The practitioners do not claim to be healers

and they do not act as intercessors. The concept is to provide support and encouragement to the individual to grow close to God in order to receive healing.

- Christian Scientists study the Bible and *Science and Health*.
- There are no ordained Clergy: weekly services are conducted by Readers who do just that, they read from the Bible and from *Science and Health*.

Naming system

Christian Science is practised worldwide, and therefore naming will reflect ethnic diversity.

Religious obligations

- Christian Scientists may observe the main Christian festivals (e.g. Christmas, Easter).
- Patients may wish to engage in private prayer, and will welcome privacy for this.

Diet

Individuals make their own decisions about diet.

Dress

This may vary depending upon the patient's country of origin.

Language

Christian Scientists will reflect the diversity of their countries of origin in their language.

Birth

In keeping with their beliefs, women will prefer to give birth with as little medical intervention as possible, unless their safety and that of their baby is at risk.

Personal hygiene

Patients will need to maintain their own high standards of cleanliness. There are no religious requirements associated with this.

Gender, privacy and dignity

- Patients will appreciate being given privacy for their prayers.
- Christian Science patients will welcome an understanding response to their wish to be treated in specific ways in accordance with their belief system.

Attitude to illness

- In general, Christian Scientists avoid hospital treatment except in the case of childbirth or in the event of an accident.
- Christian Science patients may request that drugs/therapy be kept to a minimum, as they do not believe in medical interventions.
- If hospitalised due to an accident, Christian Scientists may decline conventional medical treatment.
- Patients may request re-testing or re-evaluation prior to an impending procedure after they have had time to pray for healing.
- Patients may ask if they can contact a Christian Science practitioner – that is, a professional spiritual healer who employs the Christian Science method of healing.

Blood transfusions

Individuals make their own decisions regarding blood transfusions, although transfusions are not generally regarded as acceptable. In the case of paediatric patients some parents may agree to a blood transfusion taking place.

Contraception

Individuals make their own decisions regarding contraception.

Fertility treatment

Christian Scientists do not endorse any intervention to assist or limit conception.

Pastoral care

- Patients will welcome a visit from a Christian Science practitioner in order to receive prayer for healing.
- A worldwide directory of Christian Science practitioners is available in *The Christian Science Journal,* a monthly periodical.

Dying and death

- There are no specified last rites. Such matters remain an individual or family decision.
- Whenever possible the body of a female patient should be prepared by a female member of healthcare staff.

Autopsy

Christian Scientists will not generally support an autopsy unless there is a legal requirement for it. However, it is essential that relatives are asked about this rather than erroneous assumptions being made.

Organ and tissue donation

Individuals or their relatives make their own decisions regarding organ or tissue donation.

Jehovah's Witness

Background and beliefs

During the late nineteenth century, Charles Taze Russell, who had become disaffected with traditional Christianity within his own denomination, established a new movement, which in 1931 became known as Jehovah's Witnesses. This is a religion whose members accept the Christian Bible as the word of God and endeavour to live by the laws and principles as contained within it.

Jehovah's Witnesses consider their religion to be in line with early Christianity. They accept the Old and New Testaments of the Bible, although they do not keep the traditional festivals of the church. Witnesses do not believe that Jesus Christ is equal with God, the Father (whom they refer to as Jehovah), and they do not believe in the traditional Christian doctrine of the Holy Trinity. One holy day is kept – the death of Christ – the date of which varies as it is calculated according to Biblical formula. Witnesses believe that Christ was crucified on a stake, not a cross, as they consider the latter to be pagan. Although they remember Christ's death, they do not celebrate Easter or Christmas. They believe in Satan, considering him to be God's enemy and the cause of many of the world's problems. Witnesses do not become involved in military service or in politics, nor do they celebrate birthdays. They show a deep commitment to their faith, a major element of which is the sharing of it (witnessing) with others. A key belief of the Witnesses is in Armageddon – the holy war between Christ and Satan, during which the world will be destroyed. Because of the rather frequent occasions on which Witnesses have foretold Armageddon, they are often mocked and criticised for their beliefs and lifestyle.

One of the fundamental beliefs of Jehovah's Witnesses is that taking blood into one's body is morally wrong. Patients will not accept treatment involving the use of blood or blood products, but will accept the use of non-blood-based medical management. Jehovah's Witnesses believe that medical treatment is a matter for the informed consent of the individual.

Hospital Liaison Committees

The governing body of the Jehovah's Witnesses has created an international network of Hospital Liaison Committees in order to clarify their particular medical needs, and to gain support from medical staff in the use of bloodless procedures. Membership of the Liaison Committees consists of elders who have been specially trained to provide advice and information for doctors in relation to the provision of alternatives to blood products.

Naming system

As Jehovah's Witnesses are culturally diverse, their naming systems will vary.

Religious obligations

The only festival which is kept is that of the death of Christ, the date of which varies from one calendar year to the next.

Diet

- Because of the constraints upon the use of blood on religious grounds, some Witnesses are vegetarian.
- Witnesses who are not vegetarian will not wish to eat meat that contains blood or blood products, or meat from an animal that has been strangled, shot or not bled properly.

Dress

There are no specific issues concerning dress.

Language

This will be dependent upon the cultural/ethnic membership in a particular area.

Birth

There are no specific religious or pastoral requirements relating to birth, except in medical emergencies when the life of the mother and/or baby is at risk.

Personal hygiene

There are no specific religious requirements relating to personal hygiene.

Gender, privacy and dignity

- Witnesses are encouraged to 'keep Jehovah's organisation clean'. One of the ways in which this takes place is by members reporting the indiscretions of others to those in positions of authority.
- It is crucial that each patient is asked privately what information may be passed on to relatives.
- If a patient consents to the use of 'forbidden' blood products, there could be serious social consequences for them if this information became known.
- Healthcare staff should take extra care when discussing a Witness patient, in order to maintain privacy and confidentiality.
- Most Witnesses carry a special card identifying them as a Jehovah's Witness and releasing the hospital from responsibility in relation to the consequences of any limited treatment.

Attitude to illness

- Baptised Jehovah's Witnesses usually carry on their person an *Advance Directive/Release* document instructing that no blood transfusions should be given under any circumstances, and releasing doctors and hospitals from responsibility for any harm that might be caused by these patients' refusal of blood. This document is renewed annually.
- Many Witnesses also complete a more detailed *Healthcare Advance Directive* form that outlines their personal treatment choices with regard to blood 'fractions' and autologous blood procedures. A copy of this form is lodged with the patient's doctor.
- When Witnesses are admitted to hospital, *Release Forms* should be signed which state matters similarly and deal more specifically with the hospital care and medical alternatives to blood transfusion that will be necessary.
- Sometimes these documents can be rescinded only in writing. Difficulties may arise if a patient is well enough to rescind the decision verbally, but not in writing.

Blood transfusions

- Jehovah's Witnesses believe that allogeneic blood transfusion is prohibited by Biblical passages in both the Old and New Testaments, and are therefore opposed to taking blood or blood products on these grounds. Blood is believed to be 'the soul of the flesh' ('But you must not eat the flesh with the life, which is blood, still in it,' Genesis 9.4). In the book of Leviticus it is stated that 'The life of every living creature is the blood, and I have forbidden the Israelites to eat the blood of any creature, because the life of every creature is its blood.' In the New Testament, the Acts of the Apostles states that 'You are to abstain from meat that has been offered to idols, from blood, from anything that has been strangled.'
- Witnesses refuse all blood transfusions, including stored autologous blood.
- Witnesses refuse red cells, white cells, plasma and platelets. However, they may elect to receive fractions of these components – for example, albumin, clotting factors, immunoglobins, interferon and haemoglobin-based oxygen carriers.
- The use of the blood patch technique as a haemostatic agent is a matter of personal choice.
- Many Witnesses will accept procedures such as intra-operative blood salvage and post-operative blood salvage from drains, as well as haemodilution techniques. To make such procedures acceptable, tubing should be visible to show that the diverted blood is still in contact with the patient, as tubing is regarded as an extension of the circulatory system.
- Witnesses are able to make their own decisions in some cases – for example, in relation to bone-marrow transplants, albumin, immuno-globulin and clotting factors.
- Witnesses expect blood to be handled with respect and neither stored nor reused.
- Some Witnesses may accept dialysis if they are reassured that only their blood is being used and that the extracorporeal circulation is continuous with the body circulation.
- Any changes in blood-product policy are conveyed to Witnesses through the *Watchtower* magazine.
- The Associated Jehovah's Witnesses for Reform on Blood has been established to reform and clarify the position of the religion as a whole with regard to the use of blood and blood products.

Contraception

Married couples privately and responsibly determine whether they will use appropriate methods of family planning. Witnesses avoid methods of contraception that induce abortion.

Fertility treatment

Attitudes to this may vary depending upon the type of treatment that is being proposed. Guiding principles will be the avoidance of unnecessary termination of a pregnancy and of the use of blood or blood products in any treatments.

Pastoral care

Jehovah's Witnesses have arrangements covering all of the main hospitals to provide spiritual support and practical assistance to Witness patients during periods of hospital admission.

Dying and death

- Jehovah's Witnesses have no special rituals or practices to perform for those who are dying, nor do they have specific last rites to be administered to those *in extremis*. Patients who are terminally ill will appreciate pastoral visits from elders.
- Jehovah's Witnesses will appreciate a quiet place for prayer with the patient and relatives.
- There is no religious objection to either burial or cremation.
- There are no special requirements to be observed by medical or nursing attendants at the time of death.

Autopsy

There are no religious restrictions upon autopsies.

Organ and tissue donation

- Witnesses may not wish to donate their organs on religious grounds, namely that another person's blood would flow through them. This prohibition is suspended in relation to the donation of corneas, which would not involve a flow of blood.
- Witnesses do support organ transplantation, although surgery of this kind would need to be performed in line with the guidelines for bloodless procedures.

Mormon (Church of Jesus Christ of Latter-Day Saints)

Background and beliefs

- Founded by Joseph Smith in Fayette, New York 1838 after a series of visions.
- The key belief of the LDS Church is that they represent a restoration of the original Christian church.
- Main beliefs are set out in 13 'Articles of Faith'.
- Mormons believe that the Holy Trinity (Father, Son and Holy Spirit) are separate and distinct members of a united Godhead, though one in purpose. Each has a glorified eternal body of flesh and bone. The Holy Ghost is a separate male personage of spirit without a physical body possessing intelligence and great influence.
- The 9th Article of Faith is taken very seriously by LDS: continual revelation.
- Three key questions form the framework of their faith:
  - From where do we come?
  - Why are we here?
  - What will happen to us after death?
- Mormons believe that they are the spiritual children of God and that everyone lived as spiritual beings in a pre-earthly existence.
- Earthly life is regarded as a test to assess whether the individual is worthy to return to God after death. Death is understood as a temporary separation from loved ones.
- Family unity is of great importance. Marriages and family relationships are 'sealed' for time and eternity.
- There is strong emphasis upon healthy living (chastity, honesty, no pornography or premarital sex, foul language or gambling) and the care of the body.

Naming system

There may be some cultural variations in the use of names, but most Mormons will follow the western form of naming.

Religious obligations

Members of the church who have undergone a special temple ceremony known as the *Endowment* wear sacred undergarments. These private garments are worn at all times. They may be removed in an emergency, but must be treated with respect. Members may choose not to wear these garments while they are inpatients.

Diet

- Mormons will not consume tea, coffee or alcohol, or use tobacco or other stimulants. Hot chocolate and other chocolate drinks are acceptable.
- Members may be vegetarian or choose to eat meat sparingly.

Gender, privacy and dignity

Members of the church who wear the sacred undergarment will appreciate sensitive awareness of this among healthcare staff.

Blood transfusions

There are no religious obligations with regard to blood transfusions.

Contraception

This is a matter for the individual couple, who will usually seek guidance from the scriptures and through prayer.

Fertility treatment

LDS do not agree with artificial insemination of single women, while artificial insemination of married women from the husband is not entirely supported. However these matters tend to be left to the individuals concerned.

Stem cell research

There is no statement from the Church on this matter so far.

Dying and death

- Members of the church will expect to receive pastoral visits from representatives of the local congregation.
- Anointing with oil is common practice, with the intention of assisting in the healing of the sick person, along with the laying on of hands for healing. Patients will welcome privacy within the ward when this service takes place.
- The Sacrament (bread and water) is also brought to patients in hospital, although this is not standard practice.
- There are no specific last rites at the time of or after death. After death the deceased should be washed and dressed in a shroud.

- If the sacred garment has been worn, it must be replaced on the body after the deceased has been washed.
- Burial is preferred to cremation.
- The bishop of the church will provide pastoral support and assist with the funeral arrangements.
- The Relief Society will also assist with the practical arrangements for the funeral.
- The Church of Jesus Christ of Latter-Day Saints believes that a living being consists of two elements, namely the physical body and the spiritual body. Death causes the separation of the two elements. The spiritual body is eternal. After death, the physical body is destroyed, while the spiritual body waits for the day of resurrection.

Autopsy

There are no religious objections to autopsies.

Organ and tissue donation

There are no religious objections to organ and tissue donation. Family members are counselled and the decision is made by individuals and their families after competent medical advice has been given and confirmation received through prayer.

Rastafari

Background and beliefs

- The Rastafarian movement originated in the 1920s in Jamaica, inspired by the teachings of a Jamaican, Marcus Garvey, who worked to promote the interests of people of African descent. The movement is linked to the roots of resistance to slavery among descendants of the black African slave families, and central to it is a strong bond with Africa. As the practice of Rastafarianism can vary widely, it is difficult to provide a clear definition.
- The essential belief of Rastafarians is that Haile Selassie I is the living God of the black race. The name was taken from the now dead Emperor of Ethiopia, Selassie, known as Ras Tafari – the Lion of Judah. Ras Tafari is believed to be the new Messiah, who will lead all black people to freedom.
- The Rastafarian name for God is Jah. The Lion of Judah represents Haile Selassie, the Conqueror. It also represents the King of Kings, as the lion is the king of beasts. Rastafarians do not regard themselves as Christians, as Christ was reborn in the new Messiah – Ras Tafari. However, they accept the Old and New Testament scriptures.

- Africa, and especially Ethiopia, is considered to be the Rastafarian's heaven on earth. There is no afterlife, in contrast to Christian belief. Rastafarians believe that Jah will send the signal for the exodus back to Ethiopia, the Promised Land.
- Rastafarians believe in reincarnation, and that life is eternal.
- Followers are known by a variety of names: Rastas, Sufferers, Locksmen, Dreads or Dreadlocks, and the well known Rastafarian.
- There is a separate code of religious practice for women.
- The Rastafarian colours are red: signifying the blood of those killed for the cause of black community throughout Jamaican history; green: Jamaica's vegetation and hope for the eradication of suppression; gold: the wealth of Ethiopia; black: colour of Africans who initiated Rastafari.
- The main aim of the movement is to bring about fundamental transformation of an unjust society.

Naming system

Some Rastafarians have biblical or Ethiopian names. Old Testament names (e.g. Moses, Zephaniah) are common.

Religious obligations

- Rastafarians follow the moral principles of the Ten Commandments, but follow the ancient laws of Ethiopia.
- Many Rastafarians belong to an organisation known as the Twelve Tribes of Israel. Its philosophy is to educate the young and assist the advancement of black people and the promotion of African and Ethiopian culture.
- The Rastafarian 'Livity' (way of life) is concerned with obeying Jah and recognising Ethiopia as the New Jerusalem and a spiritual homeland.
- Most Rastafarians do not belong to a church, although many of their beliefs are linked both to Christianity and to Judaism, because Rastafarianism is understood to be highly personal.
- Rastafarians will often use the Bible for guidance. In general their belief system is not rigid.
- Emphasis is given to mysticism, within a strong framework of personal spirituality. Meetings are held to discuss issues of importance and to provide support for members.
- Believers may be associated with the Ethiopian Orthodox or Judah Coptic churches.

Holy days

- 7 January Ethiopian Christmas.
- 21 April Groundation Day: The day Haile Selassie visited Jamaica in 1966.
- 16 July Ethiopian Constitution Day: Christianity has been in Ethiopia since 330 AD. Rastafarians regards blacks as the Jews of the Bible.
- 23 July Birthday of Emperor Haile Selassie.
- 17 August Marcus Garvey's Birthday.
- 11 September Ethiopian New Year's Day: Rastafarians regard Ethiopia as their spiritual homeland to which they expect to return.
- 2 November Commemoration of the coronation of Ras Tafari as Emperor Haile Selassie, King of Ethiopia 1930.

Diet

- Many Rastafarians adhere to a system of dietary and hygiene laws that uphold and advocate a holistic lifestyle.
- Natural food that is as fresh and pure as possible is highly valued.
- Pork, predatory fish and some types of crustaceans are regarded as particularly unwholesome.
- Dairy products and refined and processed foods are avoided.
- Alcohol is rarely taken.
- Strict Rastafarians may be vegan.
- Some Rastafarians may wish to fast.

Dress

- Many Rastafarians wear their hair long and uncut in obedience to God. The dreadlocks and beard on men are regarded as a symbol of physical and moral strength and also of black pride.
- Dreadlocks symbolise the Rastafarian's roots, as well as representing the symbol of the Lion of Judah. Rastafarian women keep their heads covered during worship and when out in public places or receiving visitors.
- Some Rastafarians keep their heads covered at all times (with hairnets or scarves for women, and knitted woollen hats for men). Many Rastafarians may not agree to have their hair cut or shaved. If this is necessary it should be kept to a minimum.
- Modesty in dress is important. African influences may be seen in the fabrics and style of clothes worn.
- Hospital gowns that preserve dignity should be provided.
- Do not assume that someone is a Rastafarian on the basis of their appearance. Listen to the individual patient, as it is the individual who will inform healthcare practice.

Language

English is spoken by many Rastafarians.

Birth

- Rastafarian women will wish to give birth without excessive use of medical support, except in cases where the health of the baby or the mother is at risk.
- Breastfeeding is strongly encouraged. If bottle-feeding is necessary, women will wish to know the content of the milk and will avoid brands containing animal products.
- Circumcision is a matter of family choice.

Personal hygiene

Rastafarian patients maintain a high standard of personal cleanliness, and will wish to adhere to this in hospital.

Gender, privacy and dignity

- Hospital gowns are considered to be immodest, so the provision of more adequate covering will be appreciated.
- Women may wish to keep themselves covered at all times.
- Most female patients who require an internal examination will prefer this to be done by a female member of healthcare staff.

Attitude to illness

- The Rastafarian belief in the body's ability to heal itself may mean that a patient may be sceptical about invasive forms of medical treatment that 'interfere with God's plans.'
- Sensitivity to the patient's beliefs is important. Detailed information about the proposed treatment and all of the options available must be provided and discussed fully with the patient and their family.
- Some Rastafarians may use herbal remedies in conjunction with standard medication. Always check this in order to avoid adverse or impaired reactions to prescribed medication.

Blood transfusions

Blood transfusions may not be acceptable, so it is essential to check this with the patient or their relatives.

Contraception

Rastafarians are opposed to contraception and abortion.

Fertility treatment

Rastafarians highly value women's natural (unassisted) fertility. If a woman has difficulty in conceiving, she may therefore find it difficult to come to terms with any interventionist support.

Pastoral care

Rastafarians have a duty to visit the sick, and may do so in groups.

Dying and death

- Friends and relatives will visit and pray for a dying person.
- Sensitivity is required in order to provide appropriate spiritual care. As there is no formal structure within their organisation, an elder may approach staff with a request for the administration of last rites for the dying person.
- Some Rastafarians may wish to avoid touching a dead person, as to do so would necessitate shaving off their hair.
- There are no specific religious requirements at the time of or after death, so the body may be prepared in the usual way.
- Burial is preferred to cremation.
- There is no funeral ceremony to mark the end of life.

Autopsy

In general an autopsy is unacceptable unless there is a legal requirement for it. However, there may be exceptions to the general rule, and healthcare staff should always check with the relatives.

Organ and tissue donation

Although there are no definitive guidelines, relatives may wish to confer with the wider Rastafarian community before a decision is reached concerning organ donation and transplant.

Hindu

Background and beliefs

Hinduism is a pluralistic religion which suggests that God can be thought of and approached in a variety of ways. This teaching is central to Hinduism. It emphasises that because we are all different, the ways in which we think of and approach the ultimate reality (i.e. God) will be different.

Hinduism offers a vast variety of concepts of God. These may be divided into three categories, namely God with form and quality, God without form, and God beyond the form and the formless. Hinduism does not advocate that any one approach is better than another. The choice is a matter for the individual.

The sanctity of life is central to Hindu teaching – Ahimsa. It teaches respect for living things, including the whole of the plant and animal kingdoms.

Hindus call Hinduism 'sanata dharma' – the eternal truth or religion. Its truth is believed to have been divinely revealed, and is passed down through the ancient scriptures known as the Veda.

Hinduism does not have a single founder, holy book or authority. There is immense diversity of belief and practice within Hinduism, depending upon an individual's country of origin and their family. Emphasis is given to the individual's beliefs and obligations.

Dharma is the name given to religious pursuits. It can mean righteous living, and it may be compared to the 'cohesive force that holds society and civilisation together.'

Hindu belief emphasises that all living beings possess a soul which passes through successive cycles of birth and rebirth. Hinduism, like Buddhism, includes the idea of karma and rebirth. Each person is believed to be reborn so that the soul may be purified and eventually join the cosmic consciousness. There are important emphases placed upon collective versus individual identity, and upon purity.

Hindus believe that a person does not live in isolation from their family, social group (caste) or environment.

Traditions that apply to all Asian cultures

- Shaking hands, hugging or embracing between the sexes is avoided when meeting members of the public, but is common between members of the same sex.
- Direct eye contact should be avoided when speaking to the patient, because it is regarded as a sign of disrespect.

- Try to maintain a formal approach during conversations.
- When meeting with a couple, direct the conversation towards the male partner only, or continue speaking to whoever takes the lead in the discussion.
- When talking with a couple, avoid referring to the wife as a 'partner.'
- Do not ask for a 'Christian name' when you mean the personal name of the patient.
- In matters of diagnosis, treatment and consent, the senior elder, and sometimes the extended family, will expect to be involved.
- A female patient may be reluctant to sign a consent form without first consulting her husband or father.

Naming system

- Hindu patients are likely to have three or four names – a given or personal name, a complimentary name (the father's name or the name of a deity), and a family name or surname.
- Use the surname or family name in all patient information, together with the personal name.
- Women who marry add their husband's first name and surname or family name to their personal name.
- The word 'bhai' (brother) may be added to men's personal names when used alone.
- The words 'bhai' or 'ben' may be added to women's names.

Religious obligations

- The individual is free to worship God in many and varied ways, and may choose to worship those deities with whom he or she feels a particular affinity.
- There are no set times for prayers.
- Puja/worship may take place in a temple in front of the deities, or at home.
- Prayers can be said individually, with the family, or in a large gathering.
- A devout Hindu may say prayers (do Puja) in the morning after a shower, in the evening, and before going to bed.
- Hindus usually gather for worship on Saturday and Sunday.
- Festivals take place throughout the year, the most important one being Diwali. This is a festival of lights that takes place in October or November.

Diet

- The different regions of India each have their own dietary practices.
- Reverence for life ('Ahimsa' – mental, physical and emotional non-injury of all beings) is central to dietary practice.

- Check the dietary requirements of each individual Hindu patient.
- Some Hindus will be vegetarian.
- Most Hindus do not eat beef or pork. The cow is a sacred animal and the pig is seen as a scavenging animal whose meat is dirty.
- Some Hindus will eat eggs.
- Dairy produce is acceptable so long as it does not contain animal fat.
- Strict vegetarian Hindus will not eat off a plate or with the same utensils that have been used to serve meat. Plastic plates and cutlery should be supplied in these circumstances.
- Certain foods are classified as 'hot' or 'cold' in terms of their effect both on the body and on the emotions. Hot foods are salty, sour or high in animal protein. It is thought that they increase the body temperature and excite the emotions. Cold foods are generally sweet or bitter and are thought to lower the body temperature, calm the emotions and help the person to be strong and happy. It is believed that dietary imbalances create physical and emotional ill health.
- There are no set rules for fasting. The decision to fast is taken individually, and may also include abstaining from speaking.
- When fasting does take place, cooked foods will not be eaten but a drink may be taken. Check with the individual concerned.
- Hindu people prefer to eat using their right hand only.

Dress

- Most Punjabi women (Muslim, Sikh or Hindu) wear Shalwar-Kamees. Shalwar are baggy trousers that have narrowed ankles and are tied around the waist using a waist lace. Kamees is a long top or shirt.
- It is common for Hindu men to wear western clothing.
- Girls often wear traditional clothes at home and western clothing outside the home.
- Asian women wear the Dupatta or Chunni, consisting of two and a half yards of material draped around the top half of the body in a variety of ways, sometimes covering the head.
- The sari is also the most common form of dress for women and is worn in many different ways, depending upon the region from which the patient originates.
- Hindu women consider the wearing of jewellery to be something sacred as well as sentimental. It is passed from one generation to the next.

Language

- Many Hindus speak English in addition to their own language.
- Hindus may speak Gujarati, Hindi, Punjabi and Bengali.
- Sanskrit is the language of Hindu sacred texts and is not a conversational language.

- When an interpreter is needed, efforts should be made to find one who is familiar with the patient's own traditions and culture. It is crucial that the interpreter can be relied upon to interpret accurately and without censorship.

Miscarriage, stillbirth and neonatal death

- If miscarriage takes place before the seventh month of pregnancy, no religious rites are required, although some parents may wish for some formal recognition of the birth and death of their baby.
- Stillborn babies are usually buried rather than cremated. This principle also applies in the case of neonatal death.
- A woman may suffer considerable guilt and shame if she has more than one pregnancy loss, whether due to miscarriage or stillbirth, as the Hindu emphasis is upon a woman's fertility and ability to bear children.

Birth

- The fetus is considered to be a person from the moment of conception, so abortion is unacceptable except in emergencies.
- Hindus believe in rebirth (i.e. that the soul is reborn many times in different bodies).
- During pregnancy the mother is encouraged to read the Hindu scriptures and to meditate. These practices are believed to encourage a positive birth into this life.
- Punsavana – the fetus ceremony – takes place during the third or fourth month of pregnancy to invoke divine qualities in the infant.
- The seventh month of pregnancy is significant, as it is believed to be the month when the soul enters the body. Further prayers – Simantonnayana – are said at this stage.
- If miscarriage takes place before the seventh month there are no religious requirements. If the baby dies from the seventh month of gestation onwards, a funeral should take place.
- After birth the baby is ceremonially washed and a golden pen dipped in honey is used to write the word AUM on his or her tongue. This ceremony may be delayed until the mother and child return home. Not all Hindus will have this ceremony performed.
- The naming ceremony takes place on the tenth day after birth. The priest draws up the baby's horoscope and chooses the first letter of his or her name.
- Mothers are traditionally expected to rest for 40 days after giving birth, in order to regain their strength.
- Gifts of clothes for the new baby are acceptable.
- The birth of a boy – the first boy – is especially welcome. There is a religious and cultural preference for sons.

Personal hygiene

- Purity (Suddha) is very important within Indian culture, creating the concept of the human body as pure, perfect and a desired state of being. Physical cleanliness is linked to Suddha and leads to the meticulous practice of personal hygiene.
- Most Hindus are accustomed to having water in the same room as the toilet.
- If there is no tap or bidet, or if a bedpan has to be used, then a container of water for washing should be provided.
- Hindu patients prefer to wash in free-flowing water (e.g. a shower or a bucket of water) rather than sit in a bath.
- Women are regarded as unclean during menstruation, and will take a special shower at the end of this time.
- Washing the hands before and after a meal is expected.
- Patients will also wish to rinse out their mouths after eating.

Gender, privacy and dignity

- Hindu women prefer to be seen by female healthcare staff.
- Long gowns should be provided for women who are being prepared for X-ray or surgery.
- Hindu women and men expect to be placed in single-sex wards to avoid embarrassment.

Attitude to illness

- Hindus believe that suffering has meaning.
- Illness is thought to be punishment for wrong behaviour in a former life.
- Sometimes blessed articles of jewellery will be placed on a black string on a patient's body. This is seen as a form of protection.
- Hindus maintain a positive attitude to illness, striving to maintain hope.
- In general, Hindu patients will accept the authority of medical staff, whether male or female.
- Hindus may prefer home remedies for illness, and consequently may be slow to seek medical advice.

Contraception

- There are no specific religious rules concerning contraception, although some traditions may offer particular guidance.
- Forms of contraception that might cause irregular periods or spotting may be inappropriate in view of the religious restrictions imposed upon

menstruating women. However, it is important for medical practitioners to inform women in these circumstances that such bleeding does not fall within such religious constraints.

- In general, abortion is not supported. However, there are exceptions to this rule, especially when a woman's life is at risk.

Fertility treatment

This will be a matter for specific consideration with the couple involved. Given the emphasis upon a woman's natural fertility, and a general reluctance to terminate pregnancy, this matter may be a difficult concept for some Hindus.

Stem cell research

There is no official position on this matter.

Pastoral care

It is expected that the family will visit continually throughout a person's hospital admission. This may necessitate hospital staff considering an extension of visiting hours to meet these needs, especially at times of crisis.

Dying and death

- The patient may wish to die at home, as this has particular religious significance.
- It is important that all close family members are present. They may wish to pray at the bedside and to make sure that all religious rites take place.
- The family may wish to be actively involved in the care of the patient, and should be asked if this is their wish.
- The patient's eldest son is expected to be present before, during and after death. This pertains even when that son is a small child.
- Families who have not performed the essential rituals may become anxious about the spiritual consequences both for themselves and for the well-being of the soul of the dead patient.
- A Hindu patient or relative may request the services of a Hindu priest/ Pandit during the last stages of life to perform the following holy rites in order to assist with the transmigration of their soul at death:
  - tying a thread around the neck or wrist to bless the dying person
  - sprinkling water from the River Ganges over the person
  - placing the sacred Tulsi leaf in the mouth
  - if possible the patient may wish to be placed on the floor on a sheet or a mat, to symbolise closeness to Mother Earth, freedom from physical constraints, and the easing of the soul's departure.

- The patient may derive some comfort from the hymns and readings of the holy books. Some may wish for images or pictures, praying beads or blessings (flowers) on or near the bed.
- Some Hindus are strict about who may touch the body after death. For example, some may feel distressed if a non-Hindu touches the body.
- Close family members usually wash the body, and may request to do this on the ward. Traditionally the eldest son takes a leading role in the washing and dressing of the body.
- The eyes are closed and the legs straightened.
- The hair or beard must not be trimmed without the relatives' consent.
- Some Hindus may wish to light a clay lamp using a piece of cotton wool soaked in ghee. Others may wish to burn an incense stick in the room.
- The patient's relatives must be consulted before any of the medical staff handle the body.
- If the relatives consent to the body being touched by non-Hindus, the following conditions apply:
  - female patients should only be handled by female medical staff
  - male patients should only be handled by male medical staff.
- Jewellery, sacred threads and other religious objects should be left in place.
- The body should be covered with a plain white sheet.
- Close relatives will wish to pay their last respects while the body remains on the ward.
- The eldest son or another male relative will attend to the funeral arrangements.
- In India and elsewhere the body is cremated within 24 hours of death.
- The hospital should try to release the body as soon as possible so that the family may make arrangements for the cremation.
- Infants and young children under 5 years of age may be buried.
- The family will not cook food until the cremation/burial has taken place.

Autopsy

- Autopsies are generally regarded as unacceptable. However, there may be exceptions to this general rule dependent upon individual circumstances.
- Hindus will be anxious for the return of all organs to the body before cremation (or burial for a child under 5 years of age) in order to secure peace in the afterlife.

Organ and tissue donation

- There are many references in Hindu scriptures that support the concept of organ donation. *Daan* is the original word for donation in Sanskrit, meaning 'selfless giving.'

- Organ donation is an integral part of the Hindu way of life as guided by the Vedas.
- Scientific treatises form an important part of the Vedas. Sage Charaka deals with internal medicine, while Sage Sushruta includes features of organ and limb transplants.

Muslim

Background and beliefs

The word 'Islam' means peace and submission, implying a peaceful way of life based on submission to the will of God/Allah. The Islamic faith is followed by many Muslims throughout the world, although there is considerable diversity of belief and thought within the faith.

A Muslim may be defined as a person who accepts the Islamic way of life, and who complies with the will of God without question.

Muslims believe that Mohammed is the prophet sent by God for all humanity. They believe that the holy book, Qur'an, is the revealed book of Allah. Mecca is the birthplace of the prophet Mohammed and is a place of profound significance for all Muslims. The Ka'bah (a cubical building built by the Prophet Abraham) is in Mecca, and it is in the direction of this building that Muslims turn for their prayers.

There are five fundamental principles that are to be practised by every Muslim.

1 Belief in the oneness of God. To bear witness that there is no one worthy of worship but Allah, and that Mohammed is Allah's servant and apostle for all humanity.
2 The reciting of five daily prayers (Salat) – in the early morning before sunrise, at noon, between noon and sunset, at sunset, and at night. These prayers are obligatory and can be offered anywhere. Friday afternoon prayer is the weekly congregational prayer.
3 Fasting during Ramadan from dawn to dusk. This involves one month of abstinence from food and drink. Ramadan occurs 11 days earlier each year, and is the ninth month of the Islamic calendar. Seriously ill people, menstruating, pregnant and breastfeeding women, elderly people in poor health, and children are exempt from the fast.
4 The giving of alms (Zakat).
5 Pilgrimage to Mecca once in a lifetime.

Naming system

Since Islam spans many countries and cultures there are names and name patterns that reflect both Islamic and local cultures. However, the following points must be remembered.

1 When Muslims marry, the woman does not usually change her name.
2 Children do not necessarily have their father's name.
3 A surname or family name may not necessarily exist.

4 People of all origins may add certain titles to names to show respect (e.g. Bibi and Begum for women). Men who are especially devout may have extra religious titles added.
5 The last name is not a shared family surname. In most Muslim families each member has a different name. For example:
   - husband: Mohammed Hafiz
   - wife: Jameela Khatoon
   - sons: Mohammed Sharif and Liaquat Ali
   - daughter: Fatima Jan.

This can cause difficulties for the following reasons.

- Most records are recorded under the husband's name, and it is this name which must be asked for, irrespective of which person (husband or wife) you are addressing.
- It cannot be assumed that, for example, Liaquat Ali's father is also called Ali.
- Some families who have settled in the West may have adopted a surname, but this may not appear on any official document (passport, etc.).
- Female Muslims also have a two-part name, although neither part has religious significance.
- The first name is always a personal name, as in the western system.
- The second name can either be a title (e.g. Bano, Begum, Bibi, Khatoon, Sultana) or another personal name (e.g. Akhtar, Jan, Kausar).
- The second name should be used for the purposes of recording the patient's details formally. Because the husband's name is different, cross-referencing will be needed.

Religious obligations

To pray five times daily
Prayers may be conducted anywhere that is convenient and clean. During illness prayers may be said sitting up or lying down, so long as the chair or bed is facing Mecca. *In major illness patients are exempt from prayer.* If there is no prayer mat available, a folded sheet or a clean towel may be used instead. The patient may draw the curtains for privacy. As the prayers do not take long (10–15 minutes), this should not cause difficulties on the ward. Some Muslims wear a Ta'weez (amulet) around their neck. This is a religious article inscribed with Qur'anic verses as a protection against evil.

Cleansing
Cleansing (Wusu or Ghusal) must be performed before touching the Qur'an. It takes the form of handwashing, gargling, rinsing the mouth

and nostrils, washing the face and the arms, passing wet hands over the hair, and washing the feet. A normal wash hand basin is adequate for performing the Ablution, but the patient may need assistance if they are elderly, frail or weak.

The direction of the Quibla

Muslims must face south-east towards the Quibla/Ka'bah in Mecca. A compass helps to find the direction for prayer. A Quibla sign may be put on the wall to avoid the need for constant use of a compass.

The Holy Qur'an

This is the most important holy book for Muslims. The Qur'an should be handled only after Ablution, and must be treated with care and respect.

Ramadan

This period of fasting usually falls in the latter part of each year, although the calendar dates will vary. Muslims are permitted to eat and drink before sunrise, but must then fast until dusk. Ramadan is a period of spiritual discipline. Children are taught to pray and keep the fast when they reach adolescence.

The sick and infirm and menstruating women are not expected to fast during Ramadan. However, some patients may wish to keep the fast while in hospital. It is important to discuss the implications of fasting with the patient and/or their relatives in order to reach an agreement about this and for medical opinion to be taken seriously in cases where fasting would further damage the patient's health. During illness a person may be given a temporary or permanent exemption from the requirement to fast, especially when fasting would worsen the condition. Patients with chronic illness may be encouraged to engage in other disciplines, such as giving alms, rather than fasting.

Practical considerations include the following.

- Although the use of oral medicine is prohibited while fasting, it is possible to adjust the preparations and the dosage times so that medication may be taken outside the hours of fasting.
- Healthcare providers need to consider how the regular appointments system for patients might be adjusted to take into account the different eating, waking and sleeping patterns of most Muslims during Ramadan.
- Community practitioners could benefit from training in how to manage fasting patients in relation to medical care.

Eid

Eid-ul-fitr is celebrated immediately after Ramadan and is the festival of breaking the fast. This is the Muslim community's assertion of unity and family solidarity. It is a community and family celebration. Presents, new clothes and money are given to children.

Eid-ul-Adha is the festival commemorating the Prophet Abraham's willingness to sacrifice his son, Ismail, in obedience to God's command. This festival falls on the day after the day of Hajj.

Diet

- Lamb, beef, goat, chicken, rabbit, deer, etc. can be consumed provided that a Muslim has slaughtered these, after prayers have been said. This is Halal food.
- Pakistani Muslims are strict about eating only Halal meat.
- Pork meat, all pork products and blood are forbidden.
- Wine and other alcoholic drinks are also forbidden.
- Muslims do not eat meat or other food containing animal fats, or fats from animals which have not been ritually slaughtered.
- Fish and eggs are permitted. These must not be cooked in conjunction with pork or non-Halal meat.
- Patients may ask their relatives to bring Halal food from home, as this is more culturally appropriate.
- Some second-generation Muslims will eat Western food (e.g. vegetables, fish, rice).
- In cooking, meat or meat products such as gelatine must be avoided.
- Separate utensils for cooking and serving the Halal food are essential.

Dress

- Muslims are required to follow rules of modesty in their dress, especially in public places where the two sexes meet.
- Women are required to cover their head (the Hijab) and to wear loose clothing.
- In some traditions women also cover their faces.
- Some men may wear a small cap, especially during prayer.
- As Muslims represent many Eastern and African cultures, there is a diversity of cultural dress among Muslims.

Language

- Depending upon their country of origin, Muslims will speak a variety of different languages.
- Some Muslims will speak English alongside the language of their country of origin.
- Languages spoken by Muslims include the following:
  - Punjabi, Urdu, Pushto and Bengali

- Serbo-Croat
- Amharic (Ethiopia)
- Gujarati, Hausa and Malay
- Somali, Arabic and Hamito-Semetic (Somalia)
- Turkish and Kurdish.

Birth

Birth ceremonies include a number of elements.

- The Adhan is the Muslim call to prayer. After birth the baby is washed and the Adhan is called softly into its right ear. The Iqamat is said into the baby's left ear.
- Something sweet (a small piece of date or some honey) is placed in the baby's mouth soon after birth.
- The baby is named on the seventh day after birth.
- The baby's head is shaved on the seventh day after birth.
- All boys are circumcised.
- Islam does not sanction female circumcision.

Personal hygiene

- Islam emphasises the importance of cleanliness. Before any worship Muslims must ensure that their clothes are clean, and perform a cleansing ritual known as Ghusal or Wusu.
  - **Ghusal** is a complete body wash with clean water, and is performed after lovemaking and after menstruation.
  - **Wusu** is a partial wash with clean water, and is performed before prayer. Wusu is void after urination, defecation, passing wind or vomiting, and must be repeated.
- Muslims prefer to wash their genitals with running water after using the toilet. This is called Istinja. A jug provided for this purpose in the toilet or bathroom is appreciated.
- Muslims use their left hand for toileting and their right hand for eating, etc. This requirement must be remembered when choosing a hand for intravenous drugs. Staff must ask the patient which hand may be used.
- If a bedpan or commode is used, fresh water must be provided for cleansing.
- Although nurses and non-Muslims are allowed to wash sick people, social conventions may apply with regard to modesty, gender and body parts. It is important to ask the patient about this, as social and cultural conventions vary.

Gender, privacy and dignity

- Men are believed to be the protectors of women. It is therefore important that they are consulted about any treatment for their wives or sisters.
- Muslims take their membership of both family and the Muslim community very seriously. In some circumstances relatives may wish to consult community elders. In life-threatening circumstances, or when there is no immediate male member of the family available, a female relative may give consent.
- Muslims regard modesty in dress as extremely important.
- A man must cover his body from the navel to the knees.
- A woman is required to cover her whole body except for the feet and the hands.
- The clothing must not be tight or transparent, and must conceal the shape of the body.
- All medical gowns must respect this need for modesty (e.g. the gowns must be suitably long and completely cover the patient's body).
- Muslims prefer to be examined by medical staff of the same gender. When circumstances do not allow this, the rules can be waived. However, some Muslim women may wish a female relative or member of staff to be present during medical examinations that are conducted by a male member of the healthcare staff.
- Muslims prefer accommodation in single-sex wards or bays.
- Muslims would not usually expect to have medical information discussed directly with the patient, preferring to refer the matter to second-degree male relatives (e.g. uncles or cousins).
- Do not touch the head or hair unless for medical purposes.

Attitude to illness

- Muslims believe that nothing can take place without the consent of Allah, according to his judgment and distinction, as nothing can happen against his will.
- Illness and suffering are regarded as a means of purification, and as a punishment for wrongdoing. A period of illness is understood as providing an opportunity to make peace with one's family and community, and with God.
- Muslims believe in a life after death, when the individual will be judged. Heaven and hell form part of the judgment given by God.
- In adversity a Muslim is forbidden to despair and is required to be patient, seeking help through prayers and remembrance of Allah.
- Islam emphasises the exercising of compassion and sympathy for the terminally ill.

- Muslims may not always display emotion during times of crisis brought about by illness, or at the death of a relative.
- Muslims may be reluctant to take drugs. During Ramadan a Muslim patient may wish to receive only essential medications.
- A Muslim woman may not wish to make important medical decisions without her husband or father present.

Blood transfusions

- In general, there are no Islamic objections to blood transfusions.
- There may be exceptions, so consultation with the patient and/or relatives is important.

Religious implications of menstruation

- Muslim women are exempt from regular prayers, fasting and undertaking the Hajj during menstruation. Although sexual intercourse is forbidden at this time, other forms of physical contact between husband and wife are permitted.
- Women may be reluctant to attend a gynaecological clinic on the basis that if an internal examination takes place this may cause bleeding.
- Many Muslim women may not realise that the religious requirements do not apply when bleeding has been induced as a result of medical examination.
- By contrast, some women may visit their doctor in order to control the menstrual pattern, particularly in advance of the Pilgrimage to Mecca (Hajj). In such circumstances, oral contraceptives are provided.

Contraception

- There are varying attitudes to contraception within the Muslim community. In general the understanding is that although contraception is allowed, it is also discouraged. However, the personal autonomy of the couple is recognised, and in practice individuals will vary widely in their contraceptive practices.
- The proportion of Muslim women who use some form of contraception is lower than that among other ethnic communities.
- Any discussion must be held in confidence and discretely – never in front of visiting relatives or friends.
- The coil appears to be the contraceptive method most favoured by Muslim women, despite the increased risks of bleeding. Possible reasons for this choice include the fact that it keeps any medical contact at a low level, including the need for consultations with a male doctor.
- Some Muslim women use oral contraceptives.

- Muslims are generally less likely to terminate pregnancies on the grounds of any abnormality. However, it must not be assumed that because Islam discourages abortion, Muslim parents should not be offered any opportunity to discuss the matter further. It is important to regard the religious framework as a crucial context in which to discuss all possibilities as fully as possible with the parents.
- Abortion is not permitted except in an emergency.
- Abortion is not permitted in cases of rape or incest, as Islam emphasises the right of the child to life.
- Permitted abortion must take place before 120 days (approximately 3 months), as according to Islam the soul is breathed into the fetus after this time. This is termed 'ensoulment.'

Fertility treatment

- Within Islam, the child's rights take precedence over those of the parents. Such rights commence even before conception, and are related to the choice of a marriage partner.
- Given this context, Islam does not support fertility treatment that uses donor sperms and eggs.
- The use of the husband's sperm in artificial insemination is generally accepted.

Stem cell research

- Genetic research and engineering to alter or delete diseased genes is allowed.
- Genetic research using stem cells from products of miscarriage or surplus ova following IVF procedures is permissible.
- Human reproductive cloning is not permitted.

Miscarriage, stillbirth and neonatal death

- Not all Muslims would ascribe personhood to a fetus that is less than 24 weeks' gestation. Muslims regard the ability to breathe as indicative of life and of personhood.
- There is no religious recognition and ritual for the burial of a fetus at less than 24 weeks' gestation. However, some parents have requested the presence of a Mufti or an Imam immediately following a miscarriage.
- Fetal remains must be buried.
- Any baby that is stillborn must be given a name.
- The baby must be buried, although there is no formal religious ceremony.
- Some parents may wish photographs to be taken of the baby, although within Islam photographs or images of the human form are forbidden.

Pastoral care

- Visiting a sick relative or friend is a faith obligation and is regarded by Muslims as a virtuous act, which is greatly rewarded by God.
- A large number of people may visit a Muslim patient to pray with and for them.
- At times of crisis many people will wish to visit. It is helpful if ward staff to certain guidelines for visiting, in order to respect the needs of other patients in the area, while supporting the wish of Muslims to visit the person who is ill.

Dying and death

- Muslims understand death to be a 'marker' of the transition from one state of being to another. Rather than fearing or fighting death, Muslims are encouraged to accept death as part of the will of Allah.
- Although Islam does not support suicide or euthanasia, equally it does not support undue suffering. There is a positive attitude to the use of pain relief.
- When a Muslim patient is near death, the relatives and/or a member of the local Mosque committee should be informed.
- In ideal circumstances Muslims much prefer to be able to die at home.
- If it is not possible for the patient to return home in order to die, generous provision must be made for relatives and friends to visit him or her. It is usual for many people to visit the dying person, and ward staff must try to make adequate space available. Visitors will sit by the patient's bed and recite verses from the Qur'an, and pray for the peaceful departure of the soul.
- The time before death is important for the extending of forgiveness among family and friends.
- The patient should be turned to face Mecca and the direction of the Ka'bah (Quibla). Turn the patient on their right side, facing south-east.
- If the patient is unable to be turned, they may be placed on their back with their feet facing in a south-east direction and their head raised slightly.
- If the patient is conscious, they will be encouraged to recite the Declaration of Faith.
- When the patient dies, the recitation of the Qur'an ceases immediately.
- Relatives will wish to:
  - close the eyes of the deceased
  - turn the body to the right, and if possible towards the Quibla
  - bandage the lower jaw to the head so that the mouth does not gape
  - flex the joints of the arms and legs to stop them becoming rigid, to enable washing and shrouding.
- A complete cleansing will take place (Ghusal). Relatives may wish to do

this on the ward. Alternatively they may wait until the body is removed to their own undertakers.

- No hair or nails must be cut.
- The body will be wrapped in a Caffan. In the absence of a Caffan, a white sheet is acceptable.
- At all times the body must be covered with due regard to modesty.
- Nursing staff may fulfil the above requirements if no relatives or representatives are present. Use disposable gloves if necessary.
- The body must be released to the relatives or to the local Muslim community, who will make arrangements for the washing, shrouding and burial according to Islamic regulations.
- Any tubes, etc. or artificial limbs should be removed.
- Any incisions should be plugged to prevent or stem a flow of blood.
- Muslims do not usually bury the corpse in a coffin, but if the law or other special circumstances require it, they will not object to this.
- Burial must take place as quickly as possible.
- The relatives will be grateful for a speedy release of the body, legal requirements permitting.
- The body of a deceased woman must be handled only by female healthcare staff.
- The body of a deceased man must be handled only by male healthcare staff.
- If relatives or members of the Muslim community are not available to take charge of the body, it may be kept in the mortuary for a short time.

End of life/resuscitation

- Muslims believe that a person who has been pronounced medically brain-dead should not be kept alive artificially.
- Resuscitation is permitted, but only after careful consultation with the family. In certain circumstances resuscitation may take place for medical reasons.

Islamic living will and advance directive

- Muslims are recommended to have a 'Living Will' and an Advance Directive.
- In addition they are advised to use the services of a case manager who will be able to represent their wishes to medical staff at any point when they become unable to speak for themselves. Equally this role may be exercised by a designated member of the family.

Autopsy

- The general opinion within Islam is that autopsy examinations are not acceptable. One of the reasons given for this is that an autopsy will delay the burial of the body. Another reason is that according to Islamic belief the deceased may still be able to feel or perceive pain. In general the desecration of the body in this way is not supported.

- Where it is essential, for legal reasons, for an autopsy to take place, it is crucial that the relatives are fully consulted.
- In circumstances where it is intended that an autopsy examination will be performed for educational purposes, full consultation with the family is essential.

Organ and tissue donation

- Organ donations must not be the outcome of any compulsion or social pressures.
- Organ transplantation is permitted on the basis of saving life or alleviating pain.

American Indian/Alaska Natives

Useful to know [1-3]

American Indian (AI) and Alaska Natives (AN) are people who have their origins in any of the original peoples of North and South America who maintain tribal affiliation or community attachment.

In the 2000 Census around 2.5 million people identified themselves as belonging to these communities. Projected population increase for these groups of people is relatively low: it is expected that there will be around 5 million individuals by 2065 – 1.1% of the total population of the USA.

The majority of AN/AI people live near urban areas with 0.5% living in non-urban areas, which includes reservations.

There are 561 federally recognised AN/AI tribes, along with more than 100 other state recognised tribes. There are other tribes that are not recognised either by a state or by the federal government. Each tribe has its own culture, beliefs and practices.

In the AN/AI culture there is a long history of mistrust of government and other recognised organisations due to broken treaties and forced relocations. Only those AI who are linked with federally recognised tribes receive any healthcare benefits. These AI tend to live on reservations and in rural communities, mostly in the Western USA and Alaska. Those AN/AI peoples who make up the remaining 36% covered by the Indian Health Service (IHS) tend to live in urban non-Indian areas making it difficult for them to access the facilities of the IHS and tribal health programmes. There is a great deal of evidence illustrating that the AN/AI population experiences much ill health alongside limited healthcare choices.

Native American Medicine [4]

- Essentially Native American medicine recognises the place of Spirit – life force – known as *ni* by the Lakota and *nilch'i* by the Navajo. The individual's spirit is crucially important, so too is the spirit of the healer and the spirit of the community, the tribe, and the environment. Any healing has to take all these elements into consideration and the relationship between each and all of them.
- Native American Indians believe that we are all connected to each other and to our environment (Mother Earth, Father Sky) through the Creator known also as Great Spirit, Great Mystery or the Maker of all things above. This concept of connection is known as The Butterfly Effect.
- Great emphasis is placed upon wholeness within Native American

spirituality which is encompassing rather than selective. Key character-
istics of their relationship to health and illness and medicine stand out:
- A focus on health, healing the person and the community.
- Disease does not always have a simple explanation; outcomes are not
  always measurable.
- What can the patient and the community learn from the illness? Is
  there a message to be found within it?
- A strong emphasis upon intuition. Healing is founded on spiritual
  truths learned from nature, elders and spiritual vision.
- A healer is a counsellor and advisor.
- Native American medicine fosters confidence in the patient, self-
  awareness and inner resources to take control of their lives and
  health.
- The health history takes into account the environment as well as
  members of the family and the tribe.
- Medical intervention should result in a cure or management of the
  illness.

Causes of illness

- May have internal causes (based in feeling and state of mind).
- May have external causes such as leading an imbalanced life with too
  much excess (e.g. alcohol excess). Some causes are attributed to spirits
  while other causes are environmental.
- Illness may be caused by physical, emotional or spiritual trauma which
  lead in turn to psychological distress, or 'loss of soul' or loss of spiritual
  power.
- Some illnesses may be caused by a person breaking the 'rules for living'
  e.g. showing disrespect for people, places, animals, objects or events.

Various Native American treatments

(Some of these may continue for lengthy periods of time – i.e. usage over
months rather than weeks)

- The Sweat Lodge
- Prayer
- Burning sage or aromatic woods (smudging)
- Laying-on-of-hands
- Massage
- Counselling
- Imagery
- Fasting
- Dreaming
- Going on a Shamanic journey

Communication[5]

- The patient will see their illness not only in personal terms but in relation to their family, the community and their environment.
- The patient's sense of time may be based upon a cyclical rather than a linear pattern. Missed appointments or late attendance are common. Good practice would indicate that it's helpful to try to fit in with this concept of time-keeping in relation to the taking of medication.
- The patient may be feeling isolated as a consequence of being far away from family on the Reservation, or conversely urban AN/AI may not have any family living nearby at all. This may deepen their anxieties.
- The patient will want to discuss their medical circumstances with their family and with the tribe before any major decisions are made, so giving time for this is essential.
- Eye contact tends to be avoided so that there is no loss of soul.
- AN/AI are taught not to express pain. Storytelling is a useful means of communicating health needs, and as a means of the health practitioner to communicate with the patient.
- Giving the patient time, and quietness in which to feel more at ease, and to develop rapport are essential.
- The head and the hair are regarded as sacred so touching the head is not acceptable unless there is medical cause to do so, and after an explanation and seeking of permission.
- The hair, jewellery, and other symbolic items may have spiritual meaning and should be accorded due respect by asking the patient's permission before attempting to remove them, if this is medically necessary. These items are best kept near the patient at all times e.g. in a clear wallet.

References

1 The Office of Minority Health, US Department of Health and Minority Studies.
2 US Office of Minority Health and Health Disparities (OMHD): American and Indian Alaskan Populations.
3 US Department of Health and Human Sciences. *The Provider's Guide to Quality and Culture/American Indian.* http://erc.msh.org/ (accessed 24 August 2008).
4 Johnston L. *Native American Medicine.* www.healingtherapies.info/Native-American%20Medicine.htm (accessed 24 August 2008).
5 University of Washington Medical Center. *Culture Clues – Communicating with American Indian/Alaska Native Patient.* Culture CluesTM is a project of the Staff Development Workgroup, Patient and Family Education Committee. University of Washington Medical Center, 2004. http://depts.washington.edu/pfes/cultureclues.html (accessed 24 August 2008).

Jain

Background and beliefs

Jains do not believe in a supreme creator God, but rather they believe that the universe has always existed. They revere and worship the 24 teachers (conquerors or pathfinders) of their faith. Mahavira, who was a contemporary of the Buddha, was the last and most recent teacher, in the sixth century BC, who revived and reformulated Jainism, and is especially honoured.

The principle of Karma, which Jains teach, is that the body inhabited by a soul in its next life is determined mainly by the soul's present actions. The human state is the only one from which release from the cycle of birth and death is possible. The teachings of the Tirthankaras lead humans to spiritual release.

Ascetism, prayer and practice enable the five Jain ideals of human development. Although there are several levels of spiritual development, most Jains are lay people whose lifestyles are influenced by the Five Great Vows of Jain Monastics. Jains believe that all souls have characteristics of infinite perception, knowledge, energy and bliss. However, these capacities of the self are restricted by karma, which is responsible for perverted conduct, injustices, rebirth and transmigration. The meaning of life is to shed karma by self-effort and free the soul from its bondage so that it can live at the apex of the universe, from where there is no rebirth.

Jainism believes in the equality of all souls, irrespective of caste, belief, race or culture, and in reverence for life as a whole. Jains are encouraged to adhere to the following key principles:

- non-violence and compassion for all living creatures
- truthfulness
- not stealing
- celibacy and chastity
- non-attachment and non-ownership
- multiplicity of views.

There is a graduated pathway known as the Three Jewels that leads towards release from karma. This pathway, which is followed by both lay people and monks and nuns, consists of the following:

- right faith
- right knowledge
- right conduct.

Since Jains and Hindus have lived side by side for thousands of years, they share some common traditions and practices.

Naming system

A Jain patient is likely to have three names:

- a personal first name
- a complimentary middle name
- a family surname.

The family surname should be used on the medical records. In general it is polite to use the patient's title plus their surname, especially when addressing an elderly person.

Religious obligations

- Prayer and worship. Jains may worship at home shrines three times a day – before dawn, at sunset and at night. They may also worship at temples, or will meet in homes or in halls.
- Fasting (tapas – practices of austerity). This may involve fasting from one meal a day, or fasting for an entire day or longer.

Diet

- Jains may eat milk, curd and ghee.
- Prohibited foods include meat, fish, eggs, butter, root vegetables, figs, honey and alcohol. Some Jains may also abstain from eating garlic and onions.
- Strict Jains may not eat after sunset or before sunrise.
- When preparing or storing food, keep prohibited foods separate from Jain foods.
- Some Jains may prefer to eat with the curtains closed in order to avoid seeing other patients eating meat, etc.
- It is a good idea to ask Jain patients whether an Asian vegetarian diet is acceptable to them, or if they require special food.
- Relatives are often willing to bring in food, so long as facilities are available for storage and heating the food.
- When fasting, Jains will not take anything except boiled water during the day. Fasting may take place on the fifth and/or fourteenth day of each lunar month. Jains may also fast for a week during the festival of Paryusana-parva in August or September.

Dress

Many Jains will wear Asian clothing, maintaining physical modesty.

Language

Jains may speak Hindi and/or Urdu, as well as English. An interpreter may be required for older patients.

Birth

It is customary for a Jain woman to rest for 40 days after giving birth, although Jain patients will adapt to the rules of the hospital. The relatives assist the mother in regaining her strength following the birth, and in caring for the baby.

Personal hygiene

Some Jains may prefer water for washing after using the toilet. There are no other specific requirements.

Gender, privacy and dignity

Female patients will usually prefer a female doctor and nurse to attend them.

Attitude to illness

- Some Jains may choose to avoid certain drugs, the taking of which may break the commitment against harming any form of life (e.g. antibiotics).
- Some Jains may also be reluctant to take opiates, due to their emphasis upon endurance, self-discipline and suffering.
- Although Jain patients may rely on spiritual practices and on human support and comfort, nevertheless they will also co-operate both with medical staff and in their own medical care.

Blood transfusions

There are no objections to blood transfusions.

Contraception

There are no religious obligations placed upon Jains with regard to contraception. However, they will avoid abortion if contraception fails. It is advisable to discuss the use of the most reliable form of contraception with couples.

Stem cell research

There is no statement on this matter to date.

Pastoral care

Jain patients will welcome visits both by members of their family and by other members of their religious community. A visit by the Brahman is especially welcome.

Dying and death

- A Jain patient who is seriously ill may derive comfort from meditation, the worship of holy images, prayer beads, prayer books, and recordings of mantras and prayers.
- Jains believe that the individual should have good thoughts, with a feeling of detachment as death approaches. The prayers and other devotions are aids to this detachment.
- It is very important that the patient's family is present. This may present difficulties both with regard to space in a ward or a side room, and in relation to the needs of other patients.
- The relatives may wish to chant or to pray with the patient.
- The relatives may chant in the patient's ear, even if he or she is not conscious.
- Some Jains may wish to burn incense, in which case careful explanation of the fire safety regulations will be advisable.
- Jain patients may wish to ask for forgiveness from relatives and friends if they have harmed them either knowingly or unknowingly. Repentance, confession and penance are very strong beliefs for Jains in relation to karma.
- The patient may wish to make a donation to a charitable cause.
- When a Jain patient is elderly or very ill, or no further treatment is appropriate for them, they may choose to withdraw from the world by means of fasting. This is in order to undertake a 'holy death.' The patient may then fast for lengthy periods, reducing their food intake until only fluids are taken, and finally reducing their fluid intake. They may also refuse all medication in such circumstances.

Autopsy

Autopsy is regarded as being disrespectful to the body. However, this attitude will vary depending upon the orthodoxy of the individual's beliefs.

Organ and tissue donation

There is generally no objection to organ donation and transplants. However, it is good practice to check this information with the individual and/or their immediate relatives or next of kin.

Jewish

Background and beliefs

Judaism is based on the belief in one universal God, seen by Jews in a personal relationship. The love of God and the wish to carry out the Ten Commandments as given to Moses on Mount Sinai are embodied in the teaching of the Pentateuch (the first five books of the Old Testament).

The three elements of Judaism are as follows.

1 **God.** God exists. God is one. God is not in bodily form. God is eternal. God knows the deeds of human beings. God punishes evil and rewards good. God will send a Messiah. God will resurrect the dead.
2 **Torah.** The Torah (teaching or direction) is of divine origin. The Torah is eternally valid.
3 **Israel.** Jews must worship God alone. God has communicated through the prophets. Moses is the greatest of the prophets.

The religious precepts are simply to:

- worship one God
- carry out the Ten Commandments
- practise charity and tolerance towards other people.

The British Jewish community identifies with neither a specific country of origin nor a particular ethnic group. However, religion and culture are inextricably mixed. There is a wide variety of beliefs and attitudes, and of languages spoken.

Observant Jews have specific dietary and other religious requirements and may hold cultural beliefs about health, illness, life and death.

There are several different traditions within Judaism, each with its own particular religious observances, namely

- Orthodox
- Reform
- Conservative or Masorti.

Orthodox Judaism consists of two groups, namely the Modern Orthodox, who have integrated into society while still observing the Jewish law, and the Ultra-Orthodox, who live separately and dress in a traditional manner.

Generic practices and requirements are given below with regard to Jewish patients, with special references to a particular tradition being made as necessary.

Keeping the Sabbath
The Sabbath is central to the rhythm of Jewish individual, family and communal life, and is observed as a day of rest and peace. Saturday is believed to correspond to the seventh day, on which God rested from the task of creation. The Sabbath begins half an hour before sunset on Friday and ends at nightfall on Saturday.

During the Sabbath all Jews are forbidden to engage in any activities that can be regarded as work. Each tradition interprets this differently. For example, Orthodox Jews will not drive a car, as this involves making a spark in the engine. By contrast, Reform Jews do not consider this to be work and therefore do drive on the Sabbath.

The exception to this is in the event of an emergency, when the requirement to sustain life takes precedence over normal Jewish law.

The practical implications for the treatment of Orthodox Jewish patients can be anticipated with some careful preparation in most cases. In circumstances where life is threatened, the requirement to sustain life takes precedence.

- Reform Jews will not object to taking medication on the Sabbath, and if the condition is serious they will accept non-kosher medication.
- Surgery, tests and other procedures can be scheduled for non-Sabbath or non-holy days.
- Orthodox Jews will expect to maintain a far stricter adherence to the Jewish law.
- All medicines must be kosher (i.e. they must not contain pig products, blood or gelatine).
- The only exception to the use of kosher medicine is if there is immediate danger of death of the patient. Then the duty to save life is the overriding principle.
- If a patient is fasting on a holy day, consider injecting the medication rather than giving a pill or tablet.
- If the patient needs to take medication daily (e.g. a diabetic who uses insulin injections), this is permitted on the grounds that it is saving/sustaining a life.
- If a blood test is needed, this will be permitted on the grounds that it is necessary for health, especially in an emergency.

Naming system

The structure of Jewish names follows the pattern of one or two personal names followed by a surname or family name.

Religious obligations

- Prayer/worship. Three daily prayers are stipulated – in the morning, in the afternoon and in the evening. Communal prayer can take place anywhere, and does not require a Rabbi to officiate.

- In the Orthodox tradition, prayer can only be said when a group of 10 or more Jewish men has been convened.
- During weekday morning prayers, some Jewish men wear Tephillin (phylacteries). These are two leather boxes containing tiny scrolls from the Torah. One is tied to the forehead and the other is bound around the left arm and hand with a leather strap.
- Prayer shawls (Tallitot) may also be worn.
- The Sabbath (Shabbat) begins half an hour before sunset on Friday evening and ends with the first sighting of three stars on Saturday evening, with a blessing for the coming week.
- During Shabbat, Jews are forbidden to engage in any activities that are considered as work. However, this is interpreted in varying ways depending upon the particular Jewish tradition to which the patient belongs and whether the individual actively practises their religion in this respect.
- 'Work 'relates to creative acts, or acts which change one condition into another. For example, a fully observant (Orthodox) Jew is not allowed to switch on or turn off a light, or even to ask someone else to do it for them during Shabbat. However, the person may accept help with this if it is offered. This law also extends to travelling, which may sometimes impact upon discharge planning. Sabbath laws also extend to a prohibition on the carrying of money or gifts, or the purchase of any articles or refreshments.
- Any religious law may be transgressed if life is in danger.
- The Torah (or Pentateuch) is the most important Jewish holy book. The Jewish patient may bring a printed version for hospital use. Synagogues keep copies of the Torah on a parchment scroll which is covered by a mantle when not in use.

Festivals

- Passover/the Festival of Unleavened Bread celebrates the Exodus from Egypt by the Children of Israel. The message is about national and personal freedom. During the festival the diet is strictly 'unleavened' and kosher hospital meals will be in accordance with this practice. No bread must be consumed. Jewish patients may prefer to have food brought from home, especially on the first night when a special meal is eaten. The festival falls at around the same time as the Christian festival of Easter.
- Ten Days of Awe (or repentance for our sins) takes place in the early autumn and commences with two days of the Jewish New Year. The tenth day is the Day of Atonement, which is a solemn 25-hour fast. If a practising Jew is in hospital at this time a doctor must be consulted

regarding the fitness of the patient to undertake this fast. Seek advice from a Rabbi of the same tradition if you are unsure.

- Tabernacles (Succoth) begins five days after Yom Kippur and cannot be kept in hospital. Orthodox Jews create temporary structures outdoors in which they eat their meals, as they remember the protection of the Children of Israel by God.
- A minor festival – Chanukah (Festival of Lights) – takes place in December (sometimes close to Christmas). Candles are lit during this festival, and some patients may wish to display Chanukah lights on the ward. Work is permitted.

During the major festivals the same laws regarding work apply. However, the actual keeping of the festivals will vary depending on the tradition to which a particular Jewish person belongs.

Diet

- Jewish food laws are known as Kashrut (fitness). Food is either permitted (kosher) or forbidden (trief).
- Animals destined for consumption by Jewish people are slaughtered by a qualified Jewish slaughterer. Permitted foods are marked with a seal to show that they are kosher.
- Observant Jews are permitted to eat the following:
  - eggs
  - milk
  - kosher chicken
  - fish (not shellfish)
  - kosher beef
  - kosher lamb
  - yoghurt
  - butter
  - cheese that has no animal content
  - all fruit and vegetables.
- Observant Jews are not permitted to eat the following:
  - pork, shellfish
  - non-kosher meat
  - milk or cheese products or items at or after meat meals. These products may be eaten separately, with a time lapse between their consumption.
- Jewish patients should be informed of the availability of kosher meals. Some may not use this facility and instead choose suitable meals from the standard menu (e.g. fish or vegetarian meals).
- Observant Jews are required to keep the preparation, serving and storage of food separate from that of non-kosher foods and implements. The following practices should be maintained on the wards.

- Kosher meals should be served with disposable cutlery and should not be removed from their container, or unsealed by staff, or put on hospital plates.
- There should be no probing to test the temperature of the food.
- Separate sets of kitchen utensils should be used for meat and milk dishes.

Dress

- Some Jewish men may wear a small cap (Kappah).
- Orthodox Jewish men prefer to be bearded or will use only an electric razor (a modern circumvention of a ruling against shaving).
- Some Jewish men may wear a prayer shawl around their waist, under a jacket or outer clothing.
- Some Jewish men may also keep a phylactery (a small box containing portions of scripture) for tying around their head and left arm while praying.
- Married Orthodox Jewish women may keep their hair covered (some women wear a wig to cover their own hair).

Language

Members of Jewish families generally use English as their main language, although Yiddish and Hebrew may also be spoken. Some Jewish people may also speak other European languages.

Birth

- An Orthodox Jewish husband will not touch his wife while she is giving birth, as Jewish teaching indicates that she is unclean at this time, due to the loss of blood.
- Within the Reformed tradition this prohibition in relation to touching would not be supported.
- Baby boys are circumcised on the eighth day after birth. The operation is postponed in the event of infantile jaundice, premature birth or any other contraindications.
- The circumcision ceremony is usually performed at home, although it can take place in hospital.
- The birth of a daughter simply requires the giving of a name.
- Among Orthodox Jews, baby girls are given their name on the Sabbath after the birth, whereas boys are named after the circumcision ceremony.
- Among Reform Jews, both boys and girls have baby-blessing ceremonies, which are normally held during the Sabbath morning services in the Synagogue.

Orthodox Jewish attitudes to miscarriage and stillbirth

- Prior to 30 days' gestation a fetus is not accorded any status as a person. If there is a miscarriage, there is no religious requirement for any prayers or a funeral. Only after a fetus has reached 30 days' gestation is it considered to have had a 'breath of life', and it should then be treated as having been a living person.
- When a fetus has reached 40 days' gestation or more but has been miscarried, the tissue must be collected and buried. The parents must be consulted about their wishes for disposal. Although the fetus must be buried, cremation of the non-fetal tissue is permitted.
- While some Orthodox Jews do not give full recognition to a stillborn baby, there will be exceptions to this rule. Parents must be offered the opportunity to hold the baby. Some Orthodox men whose families are descended from the priesthood, and who are not allowed to be near dead bodies, may have to leave the room.
- The parents may wish the baby's body to be laid out in the traditional Jewish manner prior to burial. Unless the parents specify otherwise, the Jewish Burial Society must be contacted so that they may attend to the necessary arrangements.
- The mourning period (Shivah) may not be observed.

Reform Jewish attitudes to miscarriage and stillbirth

- Reform Judaism recognises that the loss of a child, at any age of gestation, can cause profound distress to the parents and to other members of the family. This tradition recognises a need to give some formal expression to their grief.
- Although no funeral will take place, it is possible for a Rabbi to conduct a simple service in the home, if the parents request this.
- Reform Judaism recognises the trauma that stillbirth causes for the parents and extended family.
- It is possible for parents to acknowledge the loss by holding a funeral. The baby is placed in its own grave following a simple funeral service that is mainly attended by the immediate family.
- A shortened period of mourning (Shivah) may also take place, followed by the erection of a headstone with the child's name inscribed on it.

Personal hygiene

Jews are expected to wash their hands and to say a prayer before eating. There are no other specific religious requirements with regard to personal hygiene.

Gender, privacy and dignity

- Jewish patients prefer to be accommodated in single-sex wards or bays.
- Orthodox Jewish women will prefer female medical staff to examine them.
- Orthodox Jewish men consider it immodest to touch women other than their wives.
- Orthodox Jewish patients may object to female Rabbis.

Attitude to illness

- In a medical emergency the Sabbath laws are set aside, as the saving of life takes precedence over the keeping of the laws.
- Jewish people treat the medical profession with respect while at the same time being prepared to ask pertinent questions related to their condition.

Blood transfusions

There are no objections to blood transfusions.

Religious implications of menstruation

- Within the Orthodox Jewish tradition, women are considered to be unclean during menstruation. Physical contact of any kind between husband and wife is prohibited at this time.
- Within the Reform tradition this prohibition does not apply, although individual adherence will vary.
- Mikveh is ritual cleansing in water, which traditionally takes place after menstruation and marks the regaining of a woman's bodily rhythm after her period. A Mikveh is a small pool that is usually located adjacent to the Synagogue.
- Within Orthodox Judaism it is expected that a woman will attend the Mikveh each month.
- Within the more liberal traditions this ritual is not obligatory, although some women may choose to adhere to it. This may be associated more with a discovery of the Jewish feminist movement and the search for female customs and rituals than with having a relationship with the traditional Jewish concept of Mikveh.

Contraception

- Almost all Jews use some method of family planning.
- Orthodox Jews favour large families and may be reluctant to use contraception. Couples may wish to consult with a Rabbi about this.

- Abortion is permitted only in emergencies, when the pregnancy presents a physical or mental risk to the woman.
- Abortion is permitted in the case of a pregnancy arising from rape or incest.
- It is preferable for the termination to take place within the first 40 days of the pregnancy.

Orthodox Jewish attitudes to fertility treatment

There is a strong religious emphasis upon a woman's fertility, with many Orthodox Jewish families being large. Where these hopes and expectations are not met, the distress experienced by the husband and wife is immense. Jewish women who ovulate early in the cycle may be at greater risk of not conceiving if they keep the law regarding the avoidance of sexual intercourse within the first 7 days following a menstrual period. In these circumstances a couple may choose to use artificial insemination during this time, rather than break the law. However, other methods for the collection of sperm and for insemination during this time may be considered. Artificial insemination using another man's sperm would be unacceptable on religious grounds. In the same way the use of donated eggs would also be unacceptable. However, IVF using the couple's own eggs and sperm may be acceptable.

Pastoral care

- Visiting of the sick is regarded as an important religious duty, and Jewish patients may receive many visitors.
- For Orthodox Jews on the Sabbath and during major festivals visiting may be more limited, unless the visitors are able to walk to the hospital.
- The Sabbath rules are lifted when a patient is dying.
- Members of the Jewish community are also happy to visit any Jewish patients who do not have family or friends in the area.
- The Jewish Visitation Committee selects and trains Jewish people for visiting the sick in hospital, and can be contacted for details of approved visitors in the locality.

Orthodox Jewish requirements during dying and death

- A dying person should not be left alone, but must have someone sitting with them at all times.
- Jewish law prohibits any active intervention that would hasten the death of a terminally ill person. Where any ethical/religious question arises in this respect, a Rabbi should be consulted.
- In Orthodox Jewish law the moving or touching of a dying person is not permitted. The giving of pain relief is permitted.

- A dying patient may wish to recite the 'Shema' or special psalms as well as a deathbed confession known as the 'Vidui'. They may appreciate being able to hold the page on which it is written.
- Some patients will wish to see their own Rabbi or the Jewish Chaplain.
- Orthodox Jews may not accept brain death as a definition of death. The traditional understanding is that the body has to be without breath or heartbeat for a short period of time, which would then make resuscitation impossible. Some Jews may wish to use a traditional method in which a feather is placed over the nose and mouth of the deceased person as a means of detecting any breath.
- Following the death the relatives may request a Rabbi, or their local synagogue, to be contacted so that the last rites may be performed.
- If these individuals cannot be contacted, healthcare staff are permitted to perform any essential procedures as follows.
  - Close the eyes and mouth.
  - Catheters, drains and tubes should be left *in situ*, as fluid contained within them is considered to be part of the body and must be kept with it ready for burial. They may be covered with gauze or bandages.
  - Open wounds must be covered.
  - Lay out the body flat, with the hands open, the arms parallel and close to the body, and the legs stretched out straight.
  - Try to make sure that someone stays with the body (if there are no relatives) until a member of the Jewish Burial Society arrives.
  - Do not wash the body, as the Jewish Burial Society will do this. It will be a ritual washing (Taharah).
  - If death occurs on the Sabbath, the body must be removed to the mortuary until the end of the Sabbath. This consideration will also apply on Jewish holy days. Some Orthodox Jews insist on keeping watch in close proximity to the body at all times, and may request that they be allowed to sit in or near the mortuary area.
  - Traditionally the body is covered with a plain white sheet and laid on the floor, with the feet pointing towards the door.
  - A lit candle may be placed near the head.
- If the relatives are present, the son (or the nearest relative) will prepare the body as described above.
- Some families may ask to keep a vigil and remain with or near the body, to pray. This may include staying near the body while it is in the mortuary. This tradition has practical origins – vachers (watchers) were used to keep the body safe from body snatchers and rodents.
- There is a mourning period of seven days following the death.
- Jewish law requires burial to take place as soon as possible after death. Any unnecessary delay must be avoided.

Reform Jewish requirements during dying and death

- Reform Jews do not prohibit the touching of a corpse by non-Jews. The ban on the touching of dead bodies by non-Jews relates to historic pagan practices of corpse mutilation. Reform Jews support the after-death care for a Jewish patient being provided by non-Jewish healthcare staff.
- The ritual washing of the body (Taharah) will be undertaken either by trained members of the Synagogue or by the Jewish Burial Society.
- Cremation is permitted within the non-Orthodox Jewish communities, and is being increasingly used for strong theological as well as environmental reasons.

Autopsy

- Orthodox Jewish law does not allow an autopsy, except in an emergency or in cases where civil law requires it. The procedure is considered to be a desecration of the body, and emphasis is given to maintaining the physical integrity of the body whatever the cost.
- If an autopsy is essential, it is good practice for the Rabbi to be able to liaise with the Coroner.
- Reform Jews permit autopsies on the grounds that medical knowledge gained from them can be of benefit in the treatment of other people.

Practical considerations with regard to autopsy for Orthodox Jews
- Place the body on a clean white cloth so that all bodily fluids escape into the cloth.
- Unnecessary damage to the body must be avoided.
- The body must not be placed face down and, if possible, it must be kept covered.
- Samples taken from the body must be as minimal as possible.
- Wherever possible, incisions should be avoided.
- After the procedure all organs must be returned to the body, in their natural location if possible.
- The cloth must also be packed into the body.

Organ and tissue donation

- Organ donation may be permitted when the organ is needed for a specific and immediate transplant.
- Jewish law does not support the donation of organs for general medical research or to an organ bank.
- In principle, Judaism supports and encourages organ donation in order to save lives. This principle can sometimes override the strong objections to any unnecessary interference with the body after death, and the requirement for immediate burial of the complete body.

Orthodox considerations with regard to organ and tissue donation
- Orthodox authorities permit organ donations only when there is a recipient who needs the organ(s) in order to survive.
- In general, Orthodox Jews support the receipt of blood, blood products, bone marrow, corneas and kidneys. In Jewish law a doctor is obliged to screen donors before using donated blood, tissue or organs.
- For some Jews it is crucial for a person to be buried with the body intact. In such circumstances organ donation would be insupportable except in the case of blood, blood products and bone marrow, all of which are replaced naturally.

Reform considerations with regard to organ and tissue donation
- The Reform tradition supports the taking of organs in cases where there is not a specific recipient, but where there would be a use for the organs in the future.
- Similarly, the use of organs that can improve the quality of life, but not save it (e.g. eyes for corneal transplants), is supported by the Reform tradition.
- The donation of organs or tissue from a living person (e.g. a lung or a kidney, or bone marrow) is also permitted only in circumstances where it would not endanger the life of the donor.
- A Jew may receive the organs/tissues of another Jew, or of a non-Jew, which will enhance or save his or her life. This would also apply to the use of non-kosher animal organs (e.g. a pig's heart) for human transplant. The overriding principle is that the saving of life is more important than the keeping of a particular law.

Pagan

Background and beliefs

Paganism is a religion in its own right, and can be traced from prehistoric times through most ancient and modern cultures. Paganism believes in a divine creative force. It is principally rooted in the old religions of Europe, although some adherents also find great worth in the indigenous beliefs of other countries. Pagans believe in the sacredness of all things.

Pagans honour the divine in all its aspects, whether male or female. The essential personification of the divine creative force focuses upon the male and female aspects – the Mother Goddess and the Father God. The Goddess represents nourishing, synthesising and intuitive aspects, and the Father God represents the fertilising, energising, analysing and intellectual capacities. Such characteristics manifest themselves throughout the created order.

Pagans do not worship the devil. Evil is regarded as an imbalance to be corrected, and not as an independent force or entity.

Pagans make use of many different Goddess and God forms as 'tuning signals' to different aspects of the essential Goddess and God. These forms vary according to cultural, geographical and personal circumstances, and are usually envisaged in perfected human form.

Pagans believe in a multi-level reality perceived as spiritual, mental (or rational), ethical, astral and physical. Each has its own laws, which are not in conflict with one another.

Pagan philosophy and worship tend to be nature based. Mother Earth is understood as being a home, for whose well-being and protection we bear a responsibility. Pagan worship rites help believers to harmonise with natural cycles, so they are usually held at the turning points of the seasons – at the phases of the sun and moon – and at times of transition in our lives.

There is a great diversity within Paganism, which reflects the range of spiritual experience. Some Pagans follow multiple Gods and Goddesses, some focus on a single Life Force of no or specific gender, while others devote themselves to a 'cosmic couple' – Lord and Lady, God and Goddess.

Most Pagans believe in reincarnation. This is viewed as being a moral force, as it emphasises that all offences against other individuals, the community or the earth, and all failure to learn lessons must be put right by each individual, and that this responsibility cannot be evaded by physical death.

Paganism's positive ethical attitude is summed up as follows: 'Do what you will, and harm no one.'

The Pagan Federation is an umbrella organisation with a membership drawn from all strands within Paganism.

Wiccan

- Wicca is the general term for the various practices and beliefs that make up contemporary Pagan Witchcraft.
- While Wicca and Witchcraft are used interchangeably there are some Pagan Witchcraft traditions that are not Wiccan.
- Wiccan is the most practised form of Paganism, which has increasing numbers of adherents.
- Religious Witchcraft is a Pagan mystery religion which venerates the Divine in nature, and worships Goddess and God.
- While the origins of Religious Witchcraft lie in pre-Christian religious traditions, folklore, folk witchcraft and ritual magic most Witches use *The Book of Shadows* (a book of rituals and spells by Gerald Brosseau Gardner) as their main resource.
- Wiccan ideas and rites have also been absorbed by the Goddess spirituality movement.

Naming system

Some Pagans have a name that they take on becoming a Pagan. However, this name is not always used in normal circumstances, so an individual may not refer to it during any hospital admission.

Religious obligations

There are no specific obligations. Many Pagans follow an eight-fold yearly festival pattern:

1 Early February – Imbolc: The celebration of the re-awakening of the earth. These celebrations include the Goddess Bride, or Brigid, the Goddess of Light and of the hearth.
2 Spring Equinox: This celebration takes place around 21 March and remembers the Goddess Oestara, a fertility goddess who crossed the land leaving tokens of fertility (eggs, and her totem animal, the hare). The Church absorbed this into its own culture and religion, keeping Easter, with traditional Easter eggs, and the Easter bunny. Some Pagans may re-enact a battle between the Oak King who rules the summer, and the Holly King who rules the winter.
3 Beltaine (May Day): This is a celebration of fertility when the young God and Goddess come together. Bonfires and May crowns characterise this festival, although some Pagans do not agree with maypoles since they regard this as a Victorian invention. Originally farmers used to drive their cattle between two bonfires to assure fertility. Sometimes couples will jump a bonfire for the same reason.
4 Summer Solstice (around 21 June): This is the time of year when the

Sun is at its strongest and the God is at the height of his rule. Some celebrate the battle of Oak and Holly, but many reserve this battle for the two equinoxes.

5 Lughnassadh: This is the feast of the God Lugh – a God of light – and takes place in early August. The festival celebrates the first fruits of the harvest. Tradition tells of the Corn Lord taking up the fears of his people into himself and becoming the willing sacrifice who gives up his life for the good of his land.

6 Autumn Equinox (around 21 September): This celebrates the end of harvest and the return battle between Oak and Holly.

7 Samhain: This is a feast of remembrance, when the veil between the worlds becomes thin and people may receive messages from their departed loved ones. This festival places emphasis upon our human mortality, as well as kindling a hope for a time of rest and recreation before rebirth.

8 Winter Solstice (around 21 December): This feast is known as Yule and celebrates the fact that the longest night is over and that the daylight will once more begin to lengthen. Traditionally it is the festival of the rebirth of the God who was conceived at Beltaine, whose father died at Lughnassadh. There is a continuous cycle of death and rebirth throughout the Pagan year which is reflected in the smaller cycles of loss/death and renewal of life in our individual lives.

Pagans usually acknowledge the phases of the moon, of which the phase of the full moon is the most important. This is followed by the dark moon (when the moon is not seen in the sky). The first and last quarters of the moon's phases are less acknowledged.

Diet

Some Pagans are vegetarians or vegans. Others fast for personal reasons. There are no religious requirements that govern diet in general.

Dress

- No specific dress is required for a Pagan.
- Most Pagans wear symbolic jewellery that relates to their particular spiritual path. Care should be taken whenever the jewellery needs to be removed for medical reasons, and it should be returned to the person as soon as possible.

Language

Paganism is culturally and ethnically diverse.

Birth

- Birth is viewed as sacred and empowering. It is possible that Pagan women may choose not to have much pain relief, seeking to manage the pain in other ways.
- Pagan women will wish to make their own informed decisions about pre- and postnatal care.
- There are no religious requirements, but individual Pagans may have particular wishes to be considered (e.g. naming ceremonies).

Gender, privacy and dignity

There are no specific needs. In general, Pagans are relaxed about medical examinations.

Attitude to illness

- Most Pagans practise complementary therapies alongside conventional medical treatments.
- Some Pagan patients may welcome a healing ritual performed for them by Pagans who are able to do this.
- Some Pagans will regard illness as a trial set by their Gods on their road to enlightenment.
- Pagans may choose to make a Living Will and will wish to be fully informed of their condition and to make shared decisions about their treatment with healthcare professionals. Some Pagans may request that there is no intervention.

Blood transfusions

There are no religious objections to blood transfusions.

Contraception

- There are no religious objections to contraception, which is a private matter for individual couples to decide. However, pregnancies are usually planned.
- Paganism emphasises women's control over their own bodies. Women take the lead in making these decisions and are supported in the choices that they make.

Fertility treatment

There is no general prohibition regarding fertility treatment and each couple will require specific attention.

Stem cell research

There is no statement on this from any of the pagan groups to date.

Pastoral care

Pagans will naturally wish for members of their Pagan community to visit them in hospital.

Dying and death

- Pagans accept dying as part of the cycle of life, and most believe in reincarnation.
- Pagan patients will wish to know when they are dying, so that they may prepare for death.
- Rituals may take the form of 'last rites' performed by one or more Pagan members to help the spirit of the dying person to go into transition peacefully.
- If the patient or their family do not have someone specific they can ask to do this, the Pagan Federation will be able to assist.
- After death there is no requirement for the body to be dressed in particular clothes, although relatives and friends may have specific requirements.
- Some families will wish to take the body home to prepare it for burial or cremation themselves, while others will employ a funeral director.

Autopsy

There are no religious objections to autopsies, although individuals may express particular preferences.

Organ and tissue donation

There are no religious objections to this, although individuals may express particular preferences.

Heathenry

Heathenry is the term to describe the religious practices of two main groups: one historical and the other modern.

The historical Heathens were peoples who inhabited Germany, Scandinavia, and Anglo-Saxon England.

Modern Heathens are reviving the old practices and giving them various names: Asatru, The Northern Tradition, Odinism, Forn Sed, Germanic Resconstructionism or just Heathenry.

Heathenry has recently been re-accorded formal religious status in Iceland.

Heathens honour a large number of gods, goddesses and other spiritual beings whom they see as existing separately from human beings. They place a high value upon the honouring of ancestors. Heathens do not cast spells or practise any form of magic nor are Heathens Witches. Unlike Pagans they do not keep to the Eight-Fold Wheel of the Year which is based on the changing seasons and the rhythms of sunrise, sunset and the moon's phases.

- Heathenry focuses on the worship of the Norse gods.
- Communities of Heathen are known a Kindreds, or Hearths.
- Norse gods are of three different types:
  - Aesir: the gods of the clan representing kingship, order and craft
  - Vanir: the gods of the earth's fertility and the forces of nature
  - Jotnar: the giant gods who are at constant war with the Aesir. They represent chaos and destruction.
- The main deities in Asatru are:
  - Odin: god of magic, poetry, riches and the dead
  - Thor: a sky god who controls the weather, and protects the community
  - Freyr: a fertility god
  - Freyja: a fertility goddess of love and beauty.
- Heathens keep the Nine Noble Virtues:
  - Courage
  - Truth
  - Honour
  - Fidelity
  - Discipline
  - Hospitality
  - Industriousness
  - Self-Reliance
  - Perseverance.

Worship and seasons

- A central ritual is a 'blot' which is a sacrifice. Modern Heathens offer items such as honey or grain-based drink to the gods.
- Followers also engage in a ritual three-round toast: a Sumbel. The first round honours the gods, the second round honours ancestors, and the third round is kept open dependent on anyone's choice for a toast.
- Blot and Sumbel form the basis of worship at rites of passage, holidays, taking of an oath, or simply asking the gods for help (rites of need).
- Religious festivals are based around the changing seasons in spring and autumn, midsummer and winter.

Ethics

- **Wyrd** is the life force connecting everything in the universe throughout time and space. Heathens believe that all their actions have far-reaching consequences. This incurs considerable responsibility for each individual which has a strong ethical element. Taking responsibility for one's actions is therefore one of the principal ethics of Heathenry.
- **Fridh** (pronounced Frith) is the maintenance of peace and harmony within a social group. Heathens take their responsibilities towards friends, family and community very seriously.
- **Honour** is also taken very seriously: lying and deceit find little place within Heathenry. In the same way oath-taking is regarded with seriousness and Heathens will not sign anything unless they are able to give their full assent to it.

Dying and death

- Some modern Heathens believe in reincarnation.
- Heathenry is more concerned with right living in the present.
- In traditional Heathenry those who died went to one of several places:
  - those who die in battle go either to Freyja's or Odin's Hall
  - those who drown go to Ran's Hall
  - those who die of natural causes go to the Hall of the goddess Hel.
- Most Heathens today regard Hel as a neutral place where they hope to be reunited with their ancestors.

Possible implications for healthcare treatment

- A Heathen patient may require very clear and full information about medication and procedures before they are able to sign their consent.
- A Heathen patient may demonstrate stoicism with regard to difficult physical symptoms.

- Heathen patients will expect support from the Kin (family) and the community during a hospital admission.
- Individual Heathen patients may require very different things (rituals, symbols etc) at the end of life dependent upon their particular tradition.

Sikh

Background and beliefs

Sikhism originated in the Punjab about 500 years ago, and was founded by Guru Nanak, who envisaged a society in which every member would work for the common good. The word 'Sikh' means discipline. Guru Nanak drew on aspects of Hinduism and Islam to create a reformist movement. He and nine other Gurus who followed him sought to set an example of living spiritually while at the same time taking an active part in the world.

Sikhs believe in one God (the eternal source of light and creator of all being) and in many cycles of rebirth. They respect the equality of all people, regardless of caste, colour, creed or sex.

Sikhism supports and encourages free belief and the pursuit of knowledge. Followers are encouraged to make the most of opportunities in life, in order to achieve union with God through truthful conduct, humility, family life, meditation and prayer. Emphasis and encouragement are given to the service of the community. This service may include the giving of money, clothing, food and shelter to those in need. Failure in this service is believed to affect the cycle of rebirth.

The spiritual message taught by Guru Nanak has three elements:

1 meditation, which now includes chanting hymns composed by the Gurus
2 honest toil – earning a living by honest means
3 sharing – giving to the poor and needy, and contributing one-tenth of one's income to good causes.

There are around 300 000 Sikhs living in the UK. One can either be born into a Sikh family or choose to become a Sikh.

- While there are no denominations in Sikhism in the USA there is a grouping focussed on language and cultural commonalities.
- The majority of Sikhs in the USA are immigrants of Indian origin, speak Punjabi and have distinct customs and dress that originated in the Punjab.
- There is another group of Sikhs – American Sikhs (also known as Healthy, Happy, Holy Organisation) – led by Yogi Harbhajan Singh.
- American Sikhs dress distinctively in all white garments. Turbans are worn by both men and women.

Naming system

- Many Sikh names are unisex, gender being differentiated by the shared middle name to illustrate the unity of all and the eradication of caste.
- All Sikh men have the second name Singh, meaning 'lion.' All Sikh women have the middle name Kaur, meaning 'princess.' These middle names must not be confused with surnames.
- Sikhs usually prefer to be called by their first name, or by their first name and middle name (Singh or Kaur). To avoid confusion in medical records, it is best to use the family name or surname.
- Young Asians follow the western practice of using only their first and last names.

Religious obligations

- As an act of faith, baptised Sikhs wear the five K's.
  1 Kesh – uncut hair. Men wear their long hair under a turban. Women wear their hair either loose or tied back. For both men and women uncut hair symbolises sanctity and a love of nature.
  2 Kangha – a wooden comb symbolising cleanliness. It is worn above the man's top-knot, and above the woman's bun or plait.
  3 Kara – a steel bangle worn on the right wrist. It symbolises strength and restraint and is a visual link with the Gurus.
  4 Kirpan – a short sword or dagger symbolising the readiness of the Sikh to fight against injustice and to protect the oppressed. It is often worn on a cotton body belt underneath the clothes.
  5 Kaccha – a particular design of unisex undershorts with a drawstring waist. It symbolises sexual morality.
- It is important to respect the Sikh patient's need to wear the five K's, unless it is necessary for them to be removed for medical purposes.
- Nowadays most Sikhs wear only the Kesh and the Kara. Many third-generation Sikhs choose to have short hair.
- Healthcare staff should consider offering an alternative head covering to male Sikh patients pre-operatively. Equally, it may not always be necessary for the male patient to be shaved pre-operatively, thereby avoiding the shaving of the beard or cutting of long hair.
- Daily prayers are said in the early morning, at sunset and before going to sleep. These prayers may be said privately, or with other Sikhs.
- Sikh patients will have a smaller version of the holy book (the Guru Granth Sahib), called the Gutka, which contains the morning and evening prayers. It is wrapped in a clean cloth and should be kept in a clean place.
- A patient who is too ill to recite the hymns or prayers should be allowed to listen to an audiotape, or to have a relative read them aloud.

Diet

- Sikhs are forbidden to eat Halal, kosher or beef. Some Sikh women may prefer to eat no meat at all.
- Sikhs prefer to eat chicken, lamb, pork and fish.
- Some Sikhs are vegetarians.
- Vegetarian Sikhs do not eat fish or eggs.
- It is important not to use the same utensils to cook for Sikhs as have been used to cook or store Halal, kosher or beef.
- There are no specific times for fasting, although some Sikhs may wish to fast when there is a full moon.
- Most Sikhs do not smoke or drink alcohol.

Dress

- Many male Sikh patients will wear a smaller version of the turban to cover their hair while in hospital.
- Removing the turban without permission, except in an emergency, is considered an insult.
- There is no restriction on what women may wear. However, female Sikhs will tend to wear Punjabi female dress consisting of loose trousers and a tunic, with a headscarf (Shalwar-Kamees and a dupatta).

Language

- Members of Sikh families may speak several languages other than English.
- In general, Punjabi is most commonly spoken by Sikhs, and sometimes Swahili. Punjabi speakers may also understand Urdu and Hindi to some extent.

Birth

- There are no religious practices associated with birth.
- Relatives will be keen to visit the mother and baby as soon as possible after the birth, bringing with them gifts of clothes for the new arrival.
- Relatives will be concerned to allow the mother complete rest for 40 days after giving birth. This attitude is based on the belief that a woman is at her weakest at this time.

Personal hygiene

- Sikhism emphasises cleanliness.
- Sikhs prefer to wash in free-flowing water. Thus showers are preferred to baths.

- Running water is needed for washing after using the toilet or bedpan.
- Sikhs prefer to brush their teeth and wash their face and hands before eating and drinking.

Gender, privacy and dignity

- Sikhism teaches that all people are equal.
- Men and women enjoy equal status within this religion.
- Culturally, women may adopt a subservient role in public.
- Within the family, the mother-in-law or the oldest woman has significant power. This may affect the choices open to younger women in the family.
- Healthcare staff should seek to reinforce the autonomy of Sikh women in any decision making.
- Sikh women prefer to be examined by female doctors. In emergencies they do not mind being examined by male doctors so long as there is a female staff member present.
- Accommodation in single-sex wards is essential.
- Hospital gowns should be of sufficient length to avoid embarrassment.

Attitude to illness

Generally speaking, members of the Sikh community are willing to accept the authority of the professional healthcare staff. However, they may be slow to seek medical advice in the first instance.

Blood transfusions

There are no objections to blood transfusions.

Contraception

- Sikhism encourages large families.
- Contraceptives are not prohibited, and most methods are acceptable.
- Termination of a pregnancy is not supported, except in cases where the mother's health is in danger.

Miscarriage, stillbirth and neonatal death

- If a late miscarriage occurs, the baby should be given to the parents for the fulfilment of the funeral rites.
- Stillborn babies and those who die in the neonatal period may be buried.

Fertility treatment

Fertility treatment is generally acceptable to Sikhs. However, there may be reluctance to use donor eggs or sperm.

Stem cell research

- There is no official position on this matter.
- Genetic engineering to cure a disease is permissible.

Pastoral care

- It is a Sikh custom for family, friends and other members of the community to visit sick relatives. This is seen to be an act of faith and part of family life. It may be helpful to allow some easing of any regulations limiting the number of people who can visit the bedside at any one time.
- Elderly patients will have particular need of visitors for moral support and reassurance.

Dying and death

- A dying Sikh may derive comfort from reciting verses, or having them recited to him or her, from the holy book (the Guru Granth Sahib).
- Patients or relatives may request the service of a Sikh priest (granthi) during the last stages of the patient's life.
- Holy water from the Gurdwara may be given to the patient to sip, or it may be sprinkled on or around the patient.
- If no relatives are present at the time of death, they should be contacted as soon as possible.
- The relatives may wish to prepare the body, but it should not be assumed that this is the case.
- Non-Sikhs are allowed to touch the body, and healthcare staff may perform the last offices.
- The five K's must be left on the body.
- The body of the deceased should be covered with a plain white sheet.
- The body must not be sent to the hospital mortuary before any relatives arrive.
- The body may be handled by hospital staff, with due regard for the patient's requirement to be touched/attended to by healthcare staff of the same gender.
- The mouth and the eyes must be closed.
- Make sure that the patient's face is clean and straightened as necessary.
- Straighten the limbs, placing the arms by the side of the body.
- Sikh faith requires that the funeral should take place as quickly as

possible after death, if there are no legal requirements for a post-mortem.

- Sikh faith and custom require cremation of the body.

Autopsy

There are no religious objections to autopsies, although Sikhs prefer the body to remain intact.

Organ and tissue donation

- Sikhs believe that life after death is a continuous cycle of rebirth, but that the physical body is not needed for this, as a person's soul is their real essence.
- Sikh philosophy and teachings place great emphasis on the importance of giving and of putting others before oneself. It also stresses the importance of performing noble deeds. Within this context there is no objection to organ and tissue donation.

Zoroastrian

Background and beliefs

Zarathushtra was a prophet who founded Zoroastrianism, and lived in Eastern Iran around 6000 BC. Zarathushtra (the Greek name is Zoroaster) proclaimed the worship of Ahura Mazda (the Wise Lord or the Lord of Wisdom), who is believed to have created a good world consisting of seven elements of creation, namely the sky, waters, earth, plants, cattle, humans and fire.

In the tenth century a group of Zoroastrians settled in India and became known as Parsis, where the majority lived in Bombay and Gujarat state.

Zarathushtra saw the world as a theatre of conflict between two opposed moral spirits – the Spirit of Goodness and the Spirit of Evil. The highest form of existence is Asha Vahishta (highest truth and righteousness). Each person possesses Vohu-Mana (the quality of the good mind). This enables people to lay hold of Asha and to see how any part of the world may deviate from this. There is a general movement from right thoughts to right actions known as the Spirit of Piety or Devotion. The three-way pattern of Zoroastrian devotion is as follows:

1 good thoughts – humata
2 good words – hukhta
3 good deeds – hvarshta.

Zoroastrians are encouraged to live life to the full while engaging in ethical, honest and charitable activities.

The consequences of right actions lead to the establishment of the ideal society, of the kingdom of heaven. The person who lives in this way achieves a state of well-being. On dying the person enters into a state of immortal bliss.

Naming system

- Each Zoroastrian has three names – a given name, the father's forename and a family name or surname that may also indicate a profession.
- When a woman marries or remarries, the middle name is changed to that of her husband.

Religious obligations

- Before prayers, Zoroastrians will wash their hands, face and other uncovered parts of their body.
- The day is divided into five periods – sunrise to noon, noon to 3.00pm, 3.00pm to sunset, sunset to midnight, and midnight to sunrise.

- The Kushti (the sacred cord) will be untied and held before a source of light.
- Two prayers are said, preferably in a prayer room, or in privacy behind closed bed curtains.

Diet

There are no restrictions concerning diet or alcohol. However, due to personal choice some Zoroastrians will not eat pork or beef, and some are vegetarian.

Dress

Zoroastrians are required to wear two items of clothing at all times.

1 Sudreh – a white sacred shirt made of muslin or cotton that symbolises purity and good deeds.
2 Kushti – a sacred cord woven from 72 threads of fine lambswool. This symbolises the 72 chapters of the Yasna (Act of Worship), and is worn over the Sudreh.

Language

- Zoroastrians belong to what is now a dispersed community, with members settling in different parts of the world. Thus they may speak any one of a number of languages as well as English.
- An interpreter may occasionally be required.

Birth

- There are no specific religious requirements with regard to the birth of a baby.
- Parsi children are admitted into the faith at a ceremony called 'Navjote', between the ages of 7 and 15 years. The Sudreh and the Kushti are put on for the first time during this ceremony.

Personal hygiene

- Running water for washing is essential, as Zoroastrians have very high standards of hygiene.
- A bowl of fresh water at the bedside is appreciated.

Gender, privacy and dignity

The same considerations apply here as for all other patients, particularly Asian patients.

Attitude to illness

Parsees (Indian Zoroastrians) have adapted to western ways and thus accept western medication and treatments.

Blood transfusions

Zoroastrians may not accept blood transfusions. Therefore it is advisable to consult the patient and/or their relatives before proceeding.

Contraception

There are no specific religious objections to contraception.

Fertility treatment

There is no general objection to fertility treatment on religious grounds. However, careful consideration should be given to couples who practice this religion.

Pastoral care

- Zoroastrian patients will welcome visits by relatives and other members of the community.
- Prayers may be said and portions of the holy book may be read aloud.

Dying and death

According to the Zoroastrian creed, at death the soul is earthbound for three days. Because of this it is necessary to begin prayers for the dead person as soon as possible.

- If there are no relatives present, another Zoroastrian must be contacted.
- The body must be washed before being dressed in white clothing.
- A special Sudreh and Kushta must be worn under the shroud, next to the skin.
- The head may be covered by a cap or a scarf.
- The family may wish to prepare the body for the funeral, but this task is usually performed by the funeral director.

- Cremation and burial are both acceptable.
- The reasons for any potential delays to the funeral must be clearly explained.

Autopsy

Religious law prohibits autopsy except for legal reasons.

Organ and tissue donation

- Orthodox Zoroastrians consider the pollution of the body to be contrary to the will of God. Within this context there are religious objections to organ and tissue donation.
- Less Orthodox Zoroastrians may take a different approach to this issue and should be consulted.

Appendix

Care of the Chinese patient

Background and beliefs

There are three main schools of philosophical and religious thought which influence Chinese philosophy and the Chinese way of life:

- Confucianism
- Buddhism
- Taoism.

Chinese people do not consider it necessary to make distinctions between the various schools of thought. Taken together these form a distinctive philosophical and value system of which the main emphasis is pragmatic – right action and behaviour – rather than upon what might be considered to be abstractions.

Chinese people may be influenced by one or more of these religions, especially at times of crisis when they may seek traditional belief systems as a means of giving expression and meaning to their experience.

However, not all Chinese people maintain active associations with Confucianism or Taoism. For many choose Buddhism while others are Christian, and a small number are Muslim.

Confucianism

Confucius (K'ung Fu-Tzu) lived in China during a time of immense change 2500 years ago. His philosophy is based upon notions of social harmony and mutual consideration. He stressed humanistic values expressed as obligations to parents and other members of the family; obedience and respect towards older people; loyalty, integrity, self-reliance, self-control, respect and consideration for others, and benevolence. He emphasised the importance of education and knowledge.

Taoism

Taoism is an ancient Chinese philosophy which has at its heart the concept of a unifying force (Tao – pronounced 'dow') or impersonal God underlying all reality. Tao simply means The Way.

For some, Taoism is a rational philosophy which also provides an ethical framework for living. For others it is a religion and has a supernatural element. Religious Taoists believe that through following The Way they will be led through life, which is subject to change and is impermanent, to a happy eternity.

Taoism in both its forms holds the beauty and perfection of nature in very high regard. Taoists believe that through meditation and a simple life it is possible to attain purity and union with the natural world. Health, harmony and balance within the individual and between the individual and their natural surroundings, and their community are profoundly important. Conflict and confrontation are to be avoided by means of positive alternatives.

Within religious Taoism there are three groups of spirits: gods, ghosts and ancestors. Each of the gods, of which there are many, has different responsibilities and powers. The gods tend to be sought out at times of need and venerated at small shrines. Incense sticks are lit and food or other symbolic offerings are left at statues.

The veneration of ancestors is a key tradition of Taoism. Ancestors are not only those who died many years before such as great-grandparents but also those who died centuries ago. In some homes there is an ancestral shrine where wooden or paper tablets are kept which have the names of family members who have died inscribed on them. Offerings of food, symbolic paper money or paper houses, as well as incense sticks are left at the shrine. These acts of veneration celebrate and remember the achievements and good deeds and memory of the ancestors as well as seeking their help and protection. This practice instils a deep sense of belonging to a family which transcends earthly and historic boundaries, as well as strengthening ties of loyalty and respect.

Alongside the veneration of ancestors is the awareness of ghosts. These ghosts are believed to be powerful, and to exert a negative influence. Belief in ghosts extends to those ancestors who feel that they have been neglected and who come to punish their descendents. It is believed that ghosts can cause illness and disasters to individuals and to entire families. At times of vulnerability they are believed to exert even more negative powers e.g. around the time of a death, or at the birth of a child. When it is thought that there is ghostly activity families may organise religious services to exorcise the ghosts.

Good and bad luck

Good and bad luck are very important concepts in Chinese culture. This extends to such things as days, times and dates considered to be auspicious or inauspicious. At times and dates considered to be inauspicious people are likely to feel more vulnerable and to seek means of protecting themselves. Some people will take these very much into account when making plans, including an anticipated hospital admission.

Within Chinese culture there is a strong association between reality, language and thought. As a consequence positive thinking is very important as a means of successfully coping with difficulties of all kinds. By contrast, dwelling on negative thoughts and feelings, and upon such things as death and dying, are believed to increase negativity, and with that, vulnerability. Some Chinese people will avoid talking about death and certain kinds of illness (e.g. cancer). They will also avoid talking about sad or unlucky things at festivals and other happy occasions.

Some numbers are also considered to be significant. The number eight is considered to be lucky as, in Cantonese, the sound of the number sounds also like the word for prosperity. By contrast the number four is regarded as being unlucky as it sounds like the word for death.

Chinese medicine: the Ch'i principle

Ch'i, Yin and Yang are core concepts in Chinese medicine in conjunction with five elements of matter that are believed to influence the functioning of the major organs and health in general. Taoism is a major influence in the development of Chinese medicine in terms of the search for and maintenance of harmony.

Ch'i is a life force which gives life to all living organisms and circulates along 14 channels – meridians – of the body. Twelve of these meridians influence and are influenced by the major organs. The distribution of Ch'i, and its strength throughout the body, is also influenced by and depends upon a balance of Yin and Yang.

Acupuncture uses the 14 meridians in order to release and promote the flow of Ch'i in the body, thus promoting healing: a restoration of harmony and balance within the individual.

By contrast with western medicine within Chinese medicine it is believed that opposites can be both complementary and conflicting. Harmony and health are only possible when these opposites are held in balance. Yin is associated with earth, night, interior, contemplative, female, cold, and death. Yang is associated with heaven, day, exterior, activity, male, heat and life. Although the forces of yin and yang are in opposition to each other, they are interdependent and complementary and hold the universe together. The interaction of yin and yang produces change, growth, and death. Imbalance can cause illness, and death.

In excess yin may cause infections, gastric problems and great anxiety whereas an excess of yang may cause dehydration, fever, irritability and edginess.

Many Chinese people may use Chinese medicine concurrent with western medicine, or when western medicine seems to be inadequate or to be too harsh or invasive. Families also tend to pass on traditional herbal remedies. In keeping with the association of yin and yang cold and damp, heat and wind are considered as major causes of illness and physical imbalances.

In practice some Chinese medicines are effective, while others may be dangerous and result in people seeking western medical treatment far too late. Sometimes the two types of treatment are in complete disharmony with each other and cause further medical problems e.g. worsening symptoms. Western medicines such as antibiotics are regarded as yang (hot) and patients may eat foods which are yin (cold) in order to counter-balance the effects of the medication.

Given the contrasts between Chinese and western medicine it is essential that patients are asked about any alternative medication or other treatments that they may be using to avoid further complications.

Naming system

The traditional Chinese naming system has a family name, followed by a two-part personal name. These names are always used together. Quite often the first part of the personal name is shared by all the children of the same sex. A woman does not change her family name when she marries but adds her husband's family name before her own. Chinese Christians may choose a Christian personal name which will come before their Chinese personal name.

Religious obligations

Chinese New Year is the most important festival in the Chinese calendar. The date is calculated according to the lunar calendar and the festival itself last 15 days with the first week being the most important. The New Year is a time for a fresh start and for family gatherings. Dragon and lion dances are performed to bring good luck to the community. Traditions abound about what people should or should not do to avoid bad luck and to secure good luck for the year ahead. A death falling within the period of this celebration is considered to be especially unlucky.

The Lantern Festival takes place in the Spring to welcome the new season and in April there is a Festival of Souls. Families visit the graves of their ancestors. Chinese Buddhists may take food offerings and burn symbolic money at the grave.

The Dragon Boat Festival takes place in June. Races are held in dragon-shaped boats and the traditional food to be eaten is dumplings. September sees the Moon Festival when Moon Cakes are eaten and the lion dance is performed. In October a harvest festival takes place at the new moon. Traditionally people go outdoors for the day to enjoy the fresh air, and there is an expectation that they will climb to a high point to avoid bad luck.

Diet

Chinese people believe that there is an intimate relationship between food and Ch'i (Life Force). When food is metabolised it becomes Ch'i either through being a cold energy force (Yin) or as a hot energy force (Yang). In illness people are encouraged to eat those foods which will help to re-establish balance and harmony within the body. Consequently most foods are categorised in relation to whether they are Yin or Yang. For example alcohol, ginger, carbonated drinks, wheat products are considered to be Yang, whereas most vegetables, milk and other dairy products, and water are considered to be Yin. In the same way different methods of cooking are also categorised according to Yang and Yin (hot and cold), e.g. boiled and steamed foods are considered to be cold, and fried foods are considered to be hot. Rice is highly valued because it is a neutral food.

Food gains in importance and significance when people are ill. Chinese people may find it difficult to eat hospital meals (which are based upon a western diet) because they will seem to lack the elements of Yin and Yang to support healing and the rebalancing of energies in the body.

Language

Cantonese and Hakka are the most common Chinese languages although there are more than 12 Chinese languages. These languages are not mutually comprehensible just as Italian and French are not mutually comprehensible although they share the same Latin roots. By contrast with the spoken language, Chinese has only one written language

Personal hygiene

Chinese people place a high value upon physical modesty and dignity, so that any physical exposure in front of strangers can be embarrassing, particularly so for older members of the community. Women tend to prefer to be attended by female healthcare and medical staff.

Physical cleanliness is tremendously important to Chinese people who may not like baths but prefer to sponge themselves with hot water.

Draughts and cold air are considered by some to bring serious illness: older people may worry about catching a chill. In the same way some may not wash their hair when they are ill regarding it as a means of catching a chill while others may not like being placed near an open window in a ward.

The family and the community

Courtesy, respect and the maintenance of social harmony are profoundly important within the Chinese community. Emotional behaviour e.g. a display of anger is unacceptable as it disturbs the balance and harmony and shows disrespect to all concerned.

Traditionally men are regarded as being responsible for the economic support of the family and are expected to make most of the important decisions. Sons and daughters-in-law are expected to take care of the older and the frail members of the family.

The family and the community are crucially important within Chinese culture and the values that these express and support equally so. Good relationships between parents and children, kindness, respect, modesty and reserve, and a consideration for others' feelings are encouraged and are of high value. Chinese people are brought up to hide their personal feelings as the revealing of these may be considered to be bad manners. The control of feelings is subservient to the maintenance of harmony and social cohesion within the family and the community.

There is immense respect for older members of the community who have gained maturity and authority. They are a symbolic and significant link between the past and the present. Older members of the family have the role of guiding and advising the family.

Some traditional Chinese people may consider it disrespectful to ask questions. Within a healthcare setting this tradition may cause problems when patients and their families are hesitant to ask crucial questions about their health and the treatments being provided.

In addition the reputation, privacy and honour of a family are profoundly important. This may sometimes lead to families struggling to care for a sick family member rather than 'lose face' by seeking outside help and intervention, with the consequent loss of privacy.

The family is the source of care and support. Many people are cared for by their family without much recourse to healthcare providers and support. The family must always be considered in all decision-making. Sometimes the family will make a decision on behalf of the patient without the patient knowing anything about it; on other occasions decisions will be made together with the patient. There may be a high expectation among family members that they will be primarily responsible for all healthcare decisions. Equally older members of the Chinese community may consider it highly inappropriate for any family problems to be discussed with external agencies. By contrast practical help may be welcomed.

The rationale for this tradition is that by allowing the family to make decisions the patient may be spared anxiety and worry, thus enabling their recovery and the rebalancing of physical and inner harmonies. This practice may extend to the exclusion of the patient from being told of the prognosis for their illness, especially if the news to be given is negative. Rather than speak about their illness the emphasis is upon communication without the use of words. For example a change in the pattern of visiting – with more frequent visits by family members – will communicate to the patient the seriousness of his/her condition.

However, now that many Chinese people have become naturalised within their adopted country of residence these traditional patterns are changing which may cause tensions between older and younger members of their families.

Dying and death

Traditional Chinese culture teaches that illness, dying and death are dangerous subjects. Chinese people may also, following the tradition of there being a strong connection between thought, language and reality, believe that talk about dying and death before they take place will bring bad luck. In the same way those who are ill may be reluctant to go to hospital as this would be a clear statement of their illness which, within the pattern of their thinking, could hasten death. It is thought that those who are ill, or dying, as well as the bodies of dead people are surrounded by a negative force which will affect others negatively.

Consequently people prefer to cleanse themselves spiritually and physically after being in contact with a dying person, especially if they have touched them. Some may believe that it is better to die in hospital rather than at home in order to spare the home from the negative forces associated with dying and death. This separation of the sick and the dying from others may extend to the family refraining from telling neighbours of their circumstances. In more extreme circumstances families may wish treatment continued, even thought there is no benefit to the patient, as a means of avoiding the negative reality that they consider death to be.

Paradoxically Chinese people also have a pragmatic approach to death and many believe that death is the gateway to a new life. Dying people are therefore supported to make 'a good death' (putting their affairs in order; making themselves ready for the journey to their new life). However there is often little expression of emotion and minimal emphasis upon any sharing of feeling by family members in keeping with the Chinese tradition of self-discipline and restraining feeling for the sake of the harmony and wellbeing of the family and the community.

Autopsy

While there is no prohibition against autopsies some Chinese people may find this difficult given the requirement to bury the body whole. Reassurance may be required by the family that the body will be complete before the burial.

Organ and tissue donation

As Chinese culture sets a requirement for the body to be buried intact there may be reluctance among some Chinese families for organ and/or tissue donation. However, individual religious beliefs (e.g Christian, Muslim, Buddhist) may play a key role in this area.

Care of the Latino patient

Useful to know[1]

- The patient's country of origin, their education and income level may influence their perception and understanding of their illness.
- The Latino patient may understand their illness as an imbalance. This imbalance may be understood in physical terms such as hot and cold or understood in terms of natural versus supernatural.
- Latino people may make a distinction between what they regard as folk illnesses and western illnesses.
- Mental illness may not be understood as an illness but rather as being weak.
- Latino people may be passive when ill and see themselves as an innocent victim.

Communication

- Latino people place a high value on relationships and will welcome time spent with them building a relationship before any medical conversation.
- Patients may avoid eye contact with people of authority as a sign of respect. Some understand eye contact as related to evil spirits. A patient may believe their illness to be the consequence of the evil eye.
- When patients are silent this may mean that they do not understand the conversation; when they nod their head this simply means that they are listening to you, and not that they agree with what is being said.
- The family is the prime source of emotional support for patients. They may believe that the patient must be totally passive during recovery from illness.
- Women may prefer physical examinations to be done by a female doctor with a female attendant in the room.

Reference

1 University of Washington, Medical Center: Patient and Family Education Center. *Culture Clues: Communicating with your Latino Patient.* Culture CluesTM is a project of the Staff Development Workgroup, Patient and Family Education Committee. University of Washington Medical Center, 1999.

Care of the Somali patient

Background and beliefs

Somalia is an Islamic state, with the long taproots of Islam stretching back many centuries. There are many Somalis now living in Europe, refugees from the violence of civil war and political turmoil in their home country. Somalis adhere closely to their faith in respect of religious practices, and family life.

In 1991 people began leaving the country to escape the hunger, rape, and death that had become widespread. Over one million people fled to neighbouring countries such as Ethiopia, Kenya, Djibouti, Yemen, and Burundi. Most stayed in large refugee camps that were established to house the Somalis. Resettlement programmes have enabled families to move to Europe: Germany, Switzerland, Finland and England.

Naming system

The Somali naming system is quite complex, not least because there is no shared family name. Many Somalis have poor literacy skills and do not always understand the need for a consistent record of health care, or any other statutory agency intervention.

Everyone has a personal name, which is given first, then followed by their father's name, and following that the name of their paternal grandfather, great-grandfather and so on. This is a paternal line which people can trace back through many generations. For general usage most Somalis use only the first two or three names while women keep their own names when they marry. This naming system means that there is no name that links children to their parents, such as a family surname. As Somalis settle in Europe the use of a single surname is increasing e.g. by using a husband's second or third name. Traditional family life has become fractured as a consequence of seeking refuge in European cities with divorce at a high level. Divorced women often use their own name.

Family and community

A complex clan and sub-clan network dominates Somali society and can be traced back for centuries. Members of the clans and sub-clans are bound together by loyalty, rights and obligations. The majority of Somalis are members of one of the five noble clans which are then divided into the sub-clans. Members of these noble clans share a common ancestry and each clan inhabits a particular part of the country. However, the civil war has shattered this traditional and agricultural way of life, with the people of the sub-clans suffering most in the upheaval and violence of recent years having no-one above them to protect them or their livelihoods. This fractionation of tribal structures and relationships has spilled over into the lives of immigrant Somalis with violence between people continuing, although on a much smaller scale.

Somali family life is patriarchal with property and lineage traced though the father. Alongside this patriarchy runs a very deep tribal loyalty with members expected to care for and to support each other. This loyalty and support continues among the émigré Somalis. The man is the head of the household and is responsible for discipline and authority as well as providing for everyone. He is also expected to protect both female family members and the social standing of the family itself. A woman's role is to attend to the home and to care for the children. By contrast with other Muslim women Somali women do not usually maintain the rule of traditional segregation from men.

Amongst the Somali Diaspora are many women whose husbands have disappeared or who have been killed in the civil war. The women have grown in independence while also experiencing considerable loneliness and isolation. When missing husbands return to the family there is often marital stress and ultimately breakdown as it proves impossible for the husband and wife to relate together under the former tribal and familial traditions.

Somali men find it hard to find work due directly to poor language and transferrable skills. Many experience depression and other mental illness, and there are high rates of suicide.

Somalis who have been tortured or who have experienced other physical and/or emotional trauma may find medical treatments and any hospital admission threatening and distressing. In addition women who have been circumcised may also be very anxious about any treatment or procedure that involves their genital area.

The 'Evil Eye'

In Somali culture there is the concept of the 'Evil Eye'. A person can give someone else an Evil Eye either purposefully or accidentally by praising them or saying other positive things about them. Somalis believe that this brings harm or illness. Comments such as saying that someone looks 'lovely' are best avoided. In the same way mothers should not be told that their babies are big as this is believed to bring on the Evil Eye. However comments such as saying that the baby is 'healthy' are not considered to be harmful.

Language

Somalis speak their own Somali language. In addition many may speak Arabic, and some may speak English and/or Italian reflecting their colonial history.

Birth

Care of the newborn baby includes such luxurious-sounding things as warm-water baths, massages with sesame oil, and gentle passive stretching of the baby's limbs. A herb known as *malmal* is applied to the umbilical cord for the first 7 days after the birth.

It is traditional for mother and baby to remain indoors for the 40 days after the birth: this is known as *afatanbah*. The mother is supported by female relatives and friends who visit, providing food. Care is taken to protect the baby from the Evil Eye by giving the baby a bracelet of string with the herb *malmal* which is believed to ward off the threat. Incense burns throughout this period to cleanse the air and defend the infant from harmful smells. At the end of this period a celebration is held at the home of a relative or friend and a naming ceremony takes place although the naming ceremony may also take place within the first 14 – 21 days. To mark this special occasion a goat is killed and prayers are said.

In Somali culture birthdays are not celebrated. By contrast the anniversary of a death is remembered.

Circumcision

Circumcision is a common practice for both men and women and is considered as rite of passage so that the person is then recognised as a fully adult member of the community. Uncircumcised people are regarded as unclean so circumcision is regarded as essential for marriage.

Male circumcision may take place at any time between birth and five years of age and is accompanied by a community celebration which involves the sacrifice of a goat.

Female circumcision, which takes place between birth and five years of age, may take a variety of forms in relation to how much genital tissue is removed.

Death

Somalis are not accustomed to being informed in straightforward terms about their prognosis and prefer a softer approach in which the seriousness of the illness is described. As death approaches a portion of the Qur'an is read out loud to the patient

Please refer to the chapter on the Muslim faith for all other aspects of care for the Muslim patient.

Care of the Vietnamese patient

Useful to know

- Vietnamese culture, language, tradition and religious beliefs varies from region to region
- Vietnamese people may understand their illness:
  - in terms of an imbalance between the opposite forces of Yin and Yang
  - as the consequence of a cause for which the traditional remedy would be medicinal herbs or folk cures
  - as a consequence of germs.
- Vietnamese people may not always complete the course of medication on the basis that western medication is too strong.
- Hospital admission and treatment may be understood as the last stopping point before death.
- The usual administrative procedures may be alien to Vietnamese patients.
- Many young women prefer to be examined by a female doctor and may also prefer a female attendant in the room at the same time. Some women may refuse to be examined at all.
- Patients may already have used folk treatments before coming to hospital. These are not harmful:
  - coin rubbing
  - skin pinching.

Communication

- Consult with the family when the illness is serious as they may wish to make the medical decisions to avoid causing anxiety to the patient.
- The spokesperson tends to be the person who speaks the best English.
- Women take on the role of the main provider at the bedside although the whole family may care for the patient.
- Vietnamese people may indicate that they have physically heard you while being reluctant to acknowledge that they have not understood you.

- Men shake hands; this is not appropriate for women.
- Respect is shown by means of a small bow and avoiding eye contact.
- Emphasis is upon emotional self-control. This may mean that physical symptoms of pain etc may not be mentioned.
- The head may be regarded as sacred among some elder or new immigrant patients so it is best to avoid touching it unless this is medically necessary.
- Asking open ended questions assists in building rapport. In the same way actively seeking the patient's permission to discuss subjects and making sure that they have understood everything builds trust.

Further reading

Akhtar S (2002) Nursing with dignity. Part 8. Islam. *Nurs Times.* **98(16):** 40–2.

Baxter C (2002) Nursing with dignity. Part 5. Rastafarianism. *Nurs Times.* **98(13):** 42–3.

Christmas M (2002) Nursing with dignity. Part 3. Christianity I. *Nurs Times.* **98(11):** 37–9.

Cobb M and Robshaw V (eds) (1998) *The Spiritual Challenge of Healthcare.* Elsevier, London.

Collins A (2002) Nursing with dignity. Part 1. Judaism. *Nurs Times.* **98(9):** 33–5.

Faith Regen UK in conjunction with Faith in London (FiL) (2002) *Faith Communities Toolkit. A resource proposed for use within Jobcentreplus.* Faith Regen UK in conjunction with Faith in London (FiL), London.

Gill BK (2002) Nursing with dignity. Part 6. Sikhism. *Nurs Times.* **98(14):** 39–41.

Jogee M and Lal S (1999) *Religions and Cultures. A guide to beliefs and customs for health staff and social care services.* Edinburgh and Lothians Racial Equality Council, Edinburgh.

Jootun D (2002) Nursing with dignity. Part 7. Hinduism. *Nurs Times.* **98(15):** 38–40.

Karmi G (ed.) (1992) *The Ethnic Health Factfile: a guide for health professionals who care for people from ethnic backgrounds.* Health and Ethnicity Programme, Edinburgh.

Lawson R (2003) *Religious and Cultural Needs.* Barnet and Chase Farm NHS Trust, Herts.

Northcott N (2002) Nursing with dignity. Part 2. Buddhism. *Nurs Times.* **98(10):** 36–8.

Orchard O (ed.) (2001) *Spirituality in Healthcare Contexts.* Jessica Kingsley Publishers, London.

Papadopoulos I (2002) Nursing with dignity. Part 4. Christianity II. *Nurs Times.* **98(12):** 36–7.

Romain J (1991) *Faith and Practice: a guide to Reform Judaism today.* Reform Synagogues of Great Britain, London.

Schott J and Henley A (1996) *Culture, Religion and Childbearing in a Multiracial Society. A handbook for health professionals.* Butterworth–Heinemann, Oxford.

Schott J and Henley A (1999) *Culture, Religion and Patient Care in a Multi-Ethnic Society. A handbook for professionals.* Age Concern Books, London.

Sheikh A and Rashid Gatrad A (eds) (2008) *Caring for Muslim Patients.* 2nd edn. Radcliffe Publishing, Oxford.

Simpson J (2002) Nursing with dignity. Part 9. Jehovah's Witnesses. *Nurs Times.* **98(17):** 36–7.

Weller P (ed.) (2001) *Religions in the UK Directory 2001–03.* University of Derby, Derby.

University of Washington Medical Center. *Culture Clues: Communicating with your Vietnamese Patient.* Patient and Family Education Series.

Resources

This chapter provides further information about cultural and spiritual diversity, faith communities and support organisations.

General

Guide to the Religions of the World; www.bbc.co.uk/worldservice/people/features/world_religions/
Commission for Racial Equality; www.cre.gov.uk
Religions in the UK, a multi-faith directory published by the University of Derby in association with the Interfaith Network for the UK. Can be purchased directly from the University of Derby, Multi-Faith Centre, Kedleston Road, Derby DE22 2GB.
Inter Faith Network for the UK, 5–7 Tavistock Place, London WC1H 9SN; www.interfaith.org.uk
Equality and Diversity; www.dit.gov.uk/er/equality
The Faithworks Campaign; www.faithworkscampaign.org
Ethnicity Online (cultural awareness in healthcare); www.ethnicityonline.net

Spiritual care

Multi-faith Group for Healthcare Chaplaincy; www.mfghc.com
National Chaplaincy Strategy ('Caring for the Spirit'); www.sysha.nhs.uk

Spirituality at work

Future Business Network; www.futurebusiness.org.uk
The Grubb Institute; www.grubb.org.uk
Spirituality at Work; www.spiritualityatwork.com
Your Soul at Work; www.job-search-career.com

Research

Picker Institute Europe (provides newsletter on improvements to services within healthcare by using patient feedback); www.pickereurope.org
Positively Diverse (provides practical advice and guidance on caring for patients from various cultural backgrounds); www.doh.gov.uk/pdfs.posdivfast.pdf
Shrine (provides essential support and networking to all NHS employers, and has produced a handbook to accompany the Positively Diverse process); www.shrine.nhs.uk

American Indian/Alaska Natives

Association of American Indian Physicians; www.aaip.org
Office of Minority Health and Health Disparities; www.cdc.gov
Indian Health Service; www.ihs.gov
Mesa Creative Arts and Healing Center; www.healing-arts.org
National Congress of American Indians; www.ncai.org
Sacred Healing Circle; www.sacredhealingcircle.org

Baha'i

Baha'i; www.bahai.us
Baha'i; www.bahai.org
National Spiritual Assembly of the Baha'is of the United Kingdom, 27 Rutland
    Gate, London SW17 1PD. Tel: 0207 584 2566.

Buddhist

Buddhist; www.buddha.net
Buddhist Chaplains Network; www.buddhistchaplainsnetwork.org
Buddhist Society; www.buddsoc.org.uk
Network of Buddhist Organisations UK, The Old Courthouse, 42 Renfrew Road,
    Kennington, London SE11 4NA. Tel: 0208 682 3442.
Friends of the Western Buddhist Order; www.fwbo.org

Christian

African Methodist Episcopal Church; www.ame-church.com
African Methodist Episcopal Zion; www.amez.org
American Baptist Churches; www.abc-usa.org
Anabaptists; www.anabaptistnetwork.org
Assemblies of God; www.ag.org
Associated Jehovah's Witnesses for Reform on Blood; www.ajwrb.org
Christian Methodist Episcopal Church; www.c-m-e.org
Christian Reformed Church; www.crcna.org
Christian Science; www.tfcs.com
Church of Christ; www.churchofchrist.usa.com
Church of England; www.c-of-e.org.uk
Church of God in Christ; www.cogic.org
Church of God of the Apostolic Faith; http://cogaf.org
Churches Together in Britain and Ireland; www.ctbi.org.uk
Churches Together in England, 27 Tavistock Square, London WC1H 9HH. Tel:
    0207 529 8141; www.churches-together.org.uk
Congregationalist; www.ucc.org
Conservative Quakers; www.quaker.us
Council of Christians and Jews; www.jcrelations.com/ccjuk
Disciples of Christ; www.disciples.org

Episcopal Church; www.ecusa.anglican.org

Ethiopian World Federation, 28–34 St Agnes Place, Kennington, London SE11 4BE. Tel: 0207 735 0905; www.home.clar.net/ewfinc/rasinfo.htm

Evangelical Friends International (Quakers); www.evangelicalfriends.org

Evangelical Lutheran Church; www.elca.org

Four Square Gospel; www.foursquare.org

Free Minds; www.freeminds.org

Friends General Conference (Quakers); www.fgc.quaker.org

Friends United Meeting (Quakers); www.fum.org

General Association of Regular Baptists; www.garbc.org

Greek Orthodox Church, Thyateira House, 5 Craven House, London W2 3EN. Tel: 0207 723 4787.

Greek Orthodox; www.goarch.org

Hospital Chaplaincies Council, Church House, Great Smith Street, London SW1P 3NZ. Tel: 0207 898 1893.

Independent Friends (Quakers); www.westernquaker.net

International Pentecostal Holiness Church; www.iphc.org

Jehovah's Witnesses, Hospital Information Services, IBSA House, The Ridgeway, London NW7 1RN. Tel: 0208 906 2211; email: his@wtbts.org.uk

Jehovah's Witness USA; http://watchtower.org

Lutheran Church Missouri Synod; www.lcms.org

Lutheran Church Wisconsin; www.wels.net

Latter Day Saints; www.lds.org , www.mormon.com

National Baptist Convention; www.nationalbaptist.com

National Missionary Baptist Convention; www.nmbca.org

Pentecostal Church of God; www.pcg.org

Presbyterian Church in America; www.pcanet.org

Presbyterian Church in the USA; www.pcusa.org

Progressive National Baptist Convention; www.pnbc.org

Quakers/Society of Friends; www.quaker.org

Rastafarian; www.rastamontimes.com

Reformed in the Mainline Tradition; www.rca.org

Religious Society of Friends (Quakers); www.quaker.org.uk

Roman Catholic; www.catholic.org

Roman Catholic Church in England and Wales, 39 Eccleston Square, London SW1V 1BX; www.catholic.ew.org.uk

Russian Orthodox; www.oca.org

Salvation Army; www.salvationarmy.org.uk

Scientology; www.scientology.org

Seventh Day Adventist Church; www.adventist.org

Southern Baptist Convention; www.sbc.net

United Church of Christ; www.ucc.org

United Methodist Church; www.umc.org

United Pentecostal Church International; www.upci.org

Watchtower News; www.watchtowernews.org

Hindu

Hindu; www.hinduamericanfoundation.net

General Hindu information; www.hinduism.co.za, www.hinduismtoday.kauai.hi.us

Hindu Council (UK), 74 Llanover Road, North Wembley HA9 7LT. Tel: 07779 583066; www.hinduforum.org

Islam

American Muslim Council; www.amcnational.org

Islam Medical Association; www.imana.org

Islam; www.Islam101.com

Muslims in America; www.projectmaps.com

Learn about Islam (Prof. Alan Godlas); www.uga.edu/islam

Muslim Council of Britain, PO Box 52, Wembley HA9 0XW. Tel: 0208 903 9024; www.mcb.org.uk

Jain

Jain; www.jaina.org

Institute of Jainology, Unit 18, Silicon Business Centre, 26–28 Wandsworth Road, Greenford UB6 7JZ. Tel: 0208 997 2300.

Judaism

Conservative Judaism; www.uscj.org

Jewish Community Online; www.jewish.com/search/family/health_and_Bioethics

Jewish Lights; www.jewishlights.com

National Center for Jewish Healing; www.jewishhealing.org

Orthodox Judaism; www.ou.org

Reform Judaism; http://urj.org

Jewish Visitation Committee, United Synagogue, 8/10 Forty Avenue, Wembley HA9 8JW. Tel: 0208 385 1855.

Jewish Burial Society; www.jbs.org.uk

United Society Burial Society. Tel: 0208 343 3456.

Jewish Community Information. Tel: 0207 543 5421.

The Board of Deputies of British Jews. Tel: 0208 543 5400.

Jewish Bereavement Counselling Service. Tel: 0208 349 0839.

Drugsline Chabad (support line for drug users, former users and their relatives). Tel: 0208 518 6470.

Miyad (Jewish crisis helpline). Tel: 08457 581 999.

Chai Lifeline Cancer Care (Jewish Cancer support service). Tel: 0208 202 2211.

Jewish Association for the Mentally Ill. Tel: 0208 458 2223.

London School of Jewish Studies, Schaller House, Albert Road, Hendon, London NW4 1TE. Tel: 0208 203 6427.

Reform Synagogues of Great Britain, The Sternberg Centre for Judaism, 80 East End Road, Finchley, London N3 2SY. Tel: 0208 349 5700; www.reform judaism.org.uk

New Age

New Age; www.newageonthenet.com
Unitarian Universalism; www.uua.org
Pagan and related traditions
Asatru (Heathenry, Germanic Paganism); www.runestone.org
Pagan; www.us.paganfederation.org
Wicca; www.wicca.timerift.net
Shamanism; www.shamanism.org
The LifeRites Group, Gwndwn Mawr, Trelech, Carmarthenshire SA33 6SA. Tel: 01994 484527; www.LifeRites.org
The LifeRites group is a UK organisation that is able to provide practical help with all rites of passage, such as baby namings, funerals (celebrations of life, non-religious funerals, spiritual ceremonies) and woodland burials.
The Pagan Federation, BM Box 7097, London WC1N 3XX; www.paganfed.demon.co.uk

Sikh

Sikh; www.sikhs.org , www.sikhnet.com, www.sikhamerican.org
Network of Sikh Organisations UK, First Floor Office Suite, 192 The Broadway, Wimbledon, London SW19 1RY. Tel: 0208 540 3974.

Zoroastria

Zoroastrian; www.fezana.org
Zoroastrians in New York; www.zagny.org
Zoroastrians in Northern California; www.zanc.org
Zoroastrian Trust Funds of Europe, Zoroastrian House, 88 Compayne Gardens, West Hampstead, London NW6 3RU. Tel: 0207 328 6018; www.ztfe.com

Further resources

Center for Spirituality and the workplace; www.smu.ca
Center for the Study of Religion in Public Life; http://pewforum.org
Hartford Institute for Religion Research; www.hartsem.edu
Psychology of Religion pages (Nielsen); www.psychwww.com/psyrelig
Society for the Scientific Study of Religion; www.sssrweb.org
Tanenbaum Center for Interreligious Understanding; www.tanenbaum.org
The Association of Religious Data Archives; www.thearda.com

The Center for Spiritual Development in Childhood and Adolescence; www.
    spiritualdevelopmentcenter.org
The George Washington Institute for Spirituality and Health; www.gwumc.org
United States Department of Health and Human Services Offices of Minority
    Health; www.omhrc.gov
University of Washington Medical Center 'Culture Clues'; http://depts.washington.
    edu/pfes/cultureclues

Healthcare chaplains

Association of Professional Chaplains; www.professionalchaplains.org
Healthcare Chaplains Ministry Association; www.hcmachaplains.org
Muslim Chaplains Association; www.muslimchaplains.org
National Association of Catholic Chaplains; www.nacc.org
National Association of Jewish Chaplains; www.najc.org

Interfaith links

BeliefNet; www.beliefnet.com
Center for Christian-Muslim Understanding; www.cmcu.georgetown.edu
Interfaith Alliance Foundation; www.interfaithalliance.org
The Islamic Society of North America; www.isna.net
The Jesuit Mission and Interreligious Dialogue; www.sjweb.org
United States Conference of Catholic Bishops Office of Ecumenical and Inter-
    religious Affairs; www.usccb.org
Harvard University: The Pluralism Project; www.pluralism.org

Index